Atlas of Sleep Medicine in Infants and Children

By

Stephen H. Sheldon, D.O.
Director, Sleep Medicine Center
Children's Memorial Hospital
Assistant Professor of Pediatrics
Northwestern University Medical School
Chicago, Illinois

Susan Riter, M.D.
Attending Physician, Sleep Medicine Center
Children's Memorial Hospital
Instructor of Pediatrics
Northwestern University Medical School
Chicago, Illinois

Mark Detrojan, R. PSG. T.
Team Leader, Sleep Medicine Center
Children's Memorial Hospital
Chicago, Illinois

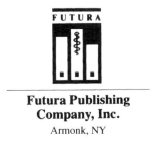

FUTURA

**Futura Publishing
Company, Inc.**
Armonk, NY

Library of Congress-in-Publication Data

Atlas of sleep medicine in infants and children / by Stephen H. Sheldon, Susan Riter, Mark Detrojan.
    p.   cm.
    Includes bibliographical references and index.
    ISBN 0-87993-423-9 (alk. paper)
    1. Sleep disorders in children—Atlases.   2. Children—Sleep—Atlases.   3. Infants—Sleep—Atlases.
4. Pulmonary function tests—Atlases.   I. Sheldon, Stephen H.   II. Riter, Susan.   III. Detrojan, Mark.
    [DNLM: 1. Sleep Disorder—in infancy & childhood.   2. Sleep Disorders—diagnosis.   3. Polysomnog-
raphy—in infancy & childhood atlases.   4. Respiratory Function Tests—in infancy & childhood atlases.
WM 188 A881 1999]
  RJ506.S55A87   1999
  618.92'8498—dc21
  DNLM/DLC
  for Library of Congress   98-37769
                                                     CIP

Copyright 1999
Futura Publishing Company, Inc.

Published by
Futura Publishing Company, Inc.
135 Bedford Road
Armonk, NY 10504-0418

ISBN #: 0-87993-423-9

Foreword

Perhaps no single area of clinical medicine has been so greatly ignored for so long as that of sleep in health and in disease. As a senior clinician, I have watched the development of sleep medicine, first as a discipline strictly limited to research laboratories, then bursting from the scientific labs into the clinical arena as a recognized specialty.

The explosion of the field of modern sleep medicine was initiated by the description of rapid eye movement (REM) sleep by Drs. Azerenski and Kleitman in the early 1950s. This was rapidly followed by observations by Drs. Dement, Kleitman, and Rechtschaffen that REM sleep was associated with dreaming. These discoveries led the way to the modern study of sleep and its disorders.

The fact that REM sleep was a "dream state" captivated the popular press and added further impetus to attract new "students" to this fledgling field. Two other significant observations added fuel. Narcolepsy syndrome, a hitherto obscure condition, was exquisitely described. It was recognized that this profound sleep-related disorder was often associated with REM sleep onset rather than with normal sleep onset through non-REM sleep. Second, Lugaresi, Duron, and others reported that some snoring patients could be apneic for as long as 80% of their total sleep time. It was simultaneously proposed that treatment and complete correction could be accomplished by simple tracheotomy. This disorder of obstructive sleep apnea syndrome and its association with daytime sleepiness became the focus of intense investigation in both scientific and clinical laboratories. As more physicians and investigators became aware of and began studying and diagnosing sleep-related disorders, it became clear that standardization within and between laboratories was required. In 1968, a standardized scoring manual edited by Drs. Rechtschaffen and Kales disciplined evaluation of sleep in both clinical and scientific laboratories. It was clear that the Rechtschaffen and Kales manual provided appropriate parameters for the evaluation of sleep in adults. Evaluating sleep in children was certainly a different matter.

In 1971, Drs. Anders, Emdee, and Parmalee provided a similar standardized scoring manual for newborn infants. Since then there has been a steady growth of knowledge of the physiology of sleep during childhood.

Research and clinical practice have advanced greatly during the last quarter of the 20th century. For example, the seminal discovery was made that narcolepsy syndrome was significantly associated with a specific HLA genotype. Not long after the identification of specific HLA antigens with narcolepsy syndrome, Lugaresi described an obscure but fatal disease associated with insomnia. This "fatal familial insomnia" was, in fact, a prion disease candidate. Chronobiology grew out of the interest of some researchers who observed that all nucleated organisms exhibited a series of oscillations of activity and inactivity with different time constants.

Pediatric sleep medicine is, indeed, in its infancy. Dr. Sheldon and colleagues have collected and presented in this atlas an impressive array of clinical data and polysomnographic observations from a large cohort of infants and children with normal and abnormal sleep. It is a valuable tool to aid the clinician in the diagnosis of all sleep-related disorders in children. Use it well!

Jean-Paul Spire, MD
Professor of Neurology and Surgery
The University of Chicago
Director, Clinical Neurophysiology and Sleep Disorders Center
University of Chicago Hospitals and Clinics

Introduction

Pediatric sleep medicine is one of the few medical disciplines still in its infancy. Although sleep disorders medicine had its start in the research laboratories of major universities throughout the world during the middle of the 20th century, clinical evaluation and treatment did not gain recognition and acceptance until the early 1980s. Indeed, clinical sleep medicine is one of the newest fields of medical art and science. At this writing there are just over 1000 certified practitioners specializing in medical disorders that have their origins during sleep. Sleep occupies more than one third of an individual's life and affects health, well-being, and performance throughout the entire 24-hour day. Practitioners of sleep medicine have been born of four basic disciplines: neurology, pulmonary medicine, psychiatry, and psychology. Very few are pediatricians.

Children are clearly different from adults, during both wakefulness and sleep. Little attention has been paid to children's sleep unless it affects the sleep of others in the family. Since children are dramatically distinct from adults, it seems reasonable that separate focus be placed on sleep of these young patients.

Similar to the development of pediatrics as a discrete medical discipline, pediatric sleep medicine has become an outgrowth of adult sleep disorders medicine. Therefore, this atlas is provided to the medical community as a beginning. It is offered to assist practitioners of this new art and science in caring for children who suffer during their hours of sleep.

Section I of this text deals with standard and recommended recording montages that may be used in the sleep laboratory. Section II presents a comprehensive discussion of pneumography, home monitoring, and event recordings. Benefits and pitfalls are discussed. Section III provides examples and discussion of recording artifacts frequently encountered during pediatric polysomnography. Finally, Section IV provides the reader with polysomnographic segments and discussion of the variety of abnormalities diagnosed and managed in the pediatric sleep disorders center.

Because of frequent repetition of specific citations for the wide variety of polysomnographic segments, selected readings and references are listed at the beginning of each section.

Abbreviations

ABD = abdominal respiratory efforts measured by piezo
    crystal belts
ALTE = apparent life-threatening event
CHEST = chest respiratory effort measured by piezo
    crystal belts
CHIN = chin muscle electromyogram (EMG)
ECG = electrocardiogram (Standard Lead 2)
EEG = electroencephalogram (Electrode placement
    according to the International 10-20 system).
EMG = electromyogram
EOG = electro-oculogram
E_tCO_2 = end-tidal carbon dioxide as measured by side
    stream capnometry (each digital representation
    of E_tCO_2 is derived from an average of the
    previous 10 seconds of air stream sampling and
    printed every second)
FLOW = nasal and oral airflow as measured by side
    stream capnography (sampling time is
    approximately 3 seconds, therefore there is a 3-
    second delay in graphic representation of the
    E_tCO_2, resulting in skewing of airflow to the
    right of chest and abdominal effort by 3
    seconds)
IMPD = chest wall impedance
LEGS = bilaterally linked anterior tibialis EMG
LOC = left outer canthus
LS = patient laying left side
MICRO = sonogram of respiratory sound recorded from
    a small microphone placed on the
    anterolateral aspect of the patient's neck
NREM = non-rapid eye movement
Pr = patient laying prone
REM = rapid eye movement
ROC = right outer canthus
R-R = R-R interval representing instantaneous heart rate
RS = patient laying right side
SaO_2/S_pO_2 = hemoglobin oxygen saturation measured
    by pulse oximetry
Su = patient laying supine
SWS = slow-wave sleep
Up = patient sitting up or body position probe off
    patient

Table of Contents

Section I

Standard and Recommended Pediatric Recording Montage

This section presents standard, recommended, and alternate polysomnographic recording montages used in evaluation of sleep and its disorders in the pediatric laboratory. Explanation of each electrode array is provided in accompanying legends. Individual epochs and discussion focusing on the reason for the specific array are also provided. In some cases, comparison of recordings are demonstrated in order to reveal the underlying basis for the choice of recommended electrode placement.

In epochs and segments where capnography was used for recording nasal and oral airflow, there is a 3-second delay (skewing) of the graphic display of airflow when compared to the display of effort. Additionally, each digital display of capnometry value for E_tCO_2 reflects an average of the prior 10 seconds of recording.

Suggested Reading

1. Anders T, Emdee A, Parmalee A: *A Manual of Standardized Terminology, Techniques and Criteria for Scoring of States of Sleep and Wakefulness in Newborn Infants.* Los Angeles: UCLA Brain Information Service, NINDS Neurological Information Network, 1971.
2. Brazier MAB: The electrical fields at the surface of the head during sleep. Electroencephalogr Clin Neurophysiol 1949;1:195–204.
3. Carskadon MA, Dement WC: The multiple sleep latency test: What does it measure? Sleep 1982;5:S67–S72.
4. Carskadon MA, Rechtschaffen A: Monitoring and staging human sleep. In Kryger MH, Roth T, Dement WC (eds): *Principles and Practice of Sleep Medicine.* Philadelphia: WB Saunders, 1989, pp. 943–959.
5. Carskadon MA, Dement WC, Mitler MM, et al: Guidelines for the multiple sleep latency test (MSLT): A standard measure of sleepiness. Sleep 1986;9:519–524.
6. Carskadon MA, Dement WC: The multiple sleep latency test: What does it measure? Sleep 1982;5:S67–S72.
7. Carskadon MA, Dement WC: Sleep tendency: An objective measure of sleep loss. Sleep Res 1977;6:200.
8. Carskadon MA, Dement WC: Sleepiness in the normal adolescent. In Guilleminault C (ed): *Sleep and Its Disorders in Children.* New York: Raven Press, 1987, pp. 53–66.
9. Carskadon MA, Harvey K, Duke P, et al: Pubertal changes in daytime sleepiness. Sleep 1980;2:453–460.
10. Clodoré M, Benoit O, Foret J, et al: The multiple sleep latency test: Individual variability and time of day effect in normal young adults. Sleep 1990;13:385–394.
11. Coble PA, Kupfer DJ, Taska LS, et al: EEG sleep of normal healthy children. Part I. Findings using standard measurement methods. Sleep 1984;7:289–303.
12. Cooper R, Osselton JW, Shaw JC: *EEG Technology.* 2nd ed. London: Butterworths, 1974.
13. Feinberg I: Changes in sleep cycle patterns with age. J Psychiatr Res 1974;10:283–306.
14. Guilleminault C: EEG arousals: Scoring rules and examples. Sleep 1992;15:173–184.
15. Jasper HH: The ten twenty electrode system of the International Federation. Electroencephalogr Clin Neurophysiol 1958;10:371–375.
16. Keenan SA: Polysomnography: Technical aspects in adolescents and adults. J Clin Neurophysiol 1992;9:21–31.
17. Keenan SA: Polysomnographic technique—An overview. In Chokroverty S (ed): *Sleep Disorders Medicine: Basic Sci-*

ence, Technical Considerations, and Clinical Aspects. Stoneham MA: Butterworth-Heinemann, 1994, pp. 79–94.

18. Rechtschaffen A, Kales A: *A Manual of Standardized Terminology: Techniques and Scoring System for Sleep Stages of Human Subjects*. Los Angeles: UCLA Brain Information Service/Brain Research Institute, 1968.

19. Ross JJ, Agnew HW Jr, Williams RL, et al: Sleep patterns in preadolescent children: An EEG-EOG study. Pediatrics 1968;42:324–335.

20. Sheldon SH: *Evaluating Sleep in Infants and Children*. Philadelphia: Lippincott-Raven, 1996.

21. Sheldon SH, Irbe D, Applebaum J, et al: Sleep pressure in children with attentional deficits. Sleep Res 1991;20A:448.

22. Walczak T, Chokroverty S: Electroencephalography, electromyography and electrooculography: General principles and basic technology. In Chokroverty S (ed): *Sleep Disorders Medicine: Basic Science, Technical Considerations, and Clinical Aspects*. Stoneham MA: Butterworth-Heinemann, 1994, pp. 95–115.

23. Williams RL, Karacan I, Hursch CJ: *Electroencephalography (EEG) of Human Sleep: Clinical Applications*. New York: Wiley, 1974.

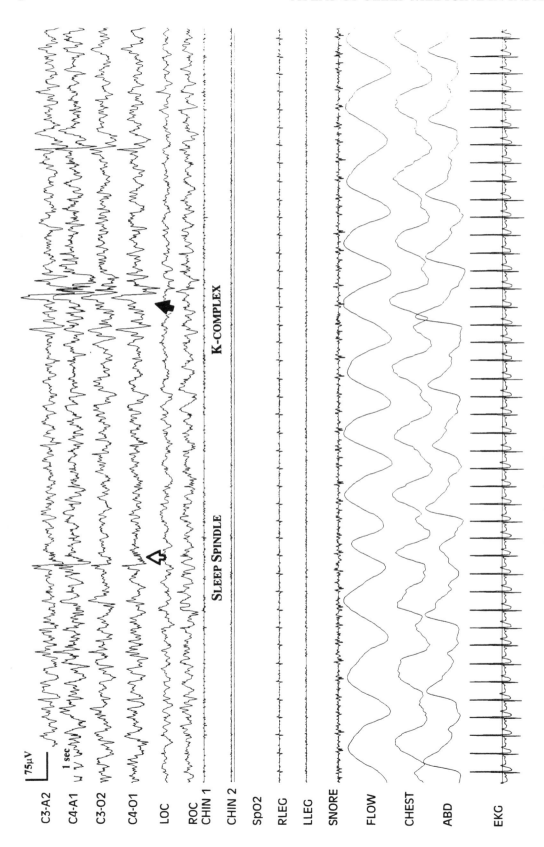

Standard Polysomnogram Montage

Figure 1. Standard Polysomnogram Montage

This polysomnographic segment demonstrates a standard recording montage used by most sleep laboratories. It consists of two central and two occipital referential channels. This EEG array is used for scoring and staging sleep. Sometimes only one central and one occipital channel are used for this purpose. EOG and Chin EMG provide the remaining channels required for sleep staging. Anterior tibialis is linked bilaterally and provides monitoring for periodic limb movements of sleep (PLMS). Some laboratories separate left leg and right leg on different channels. EKG is typically lead 2.

In this segment, nasal and oral airflow is recorded by thermistry, chest and abdominal effort is recorded by piezo crystal belts, and hemoglobin oxygen saturation is recorded by pulse oximetry.

This recording montage can provide excellent information regarding sleep state and respiration in adults. Omission of important data can, however, occur when evaluating comprehensive physiological changes during sleep in children. This youngster is in stage 2 sleep. Note sleep spindles and K complexes apparent in the EEG. EOG reveals no eye movements, EMG is tonic, and EKG reveals normal respiratory effort are monotonously regular. Both chest and abdominal efforts are in phase, and oxygen saturation is 98%.

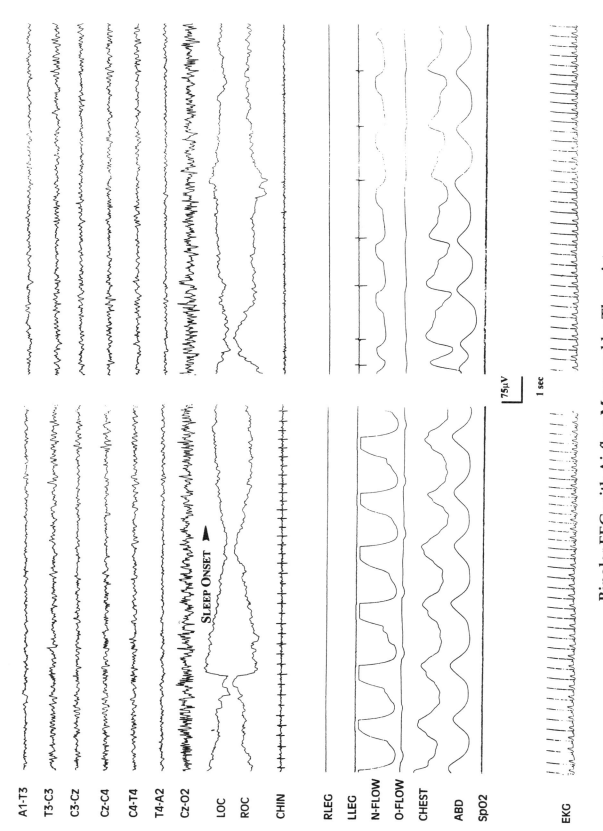

75μV

1 sec

Bipolar EEG with Airflow Measured by Thermistry

Figure 2. Bipolar EEG with Airflow Measured by Thermistry

These polysomnographic segments were recorded from a 9-year-old male being evaluated for possible sleep-disordered breathing. EEG electrode array demonstrates a bipolar trans-coronal chain extending from behind the left ear (A1) across the top of the head, through the vertex, to behind the right ear (A2). Occipital EEG activity is recorded from Cz to O2. This can also provide a referential channel for scoring sleep. Panel A demonstrates transition from wake to stage 1 sleep. Panel B demonstrates REM sleep.

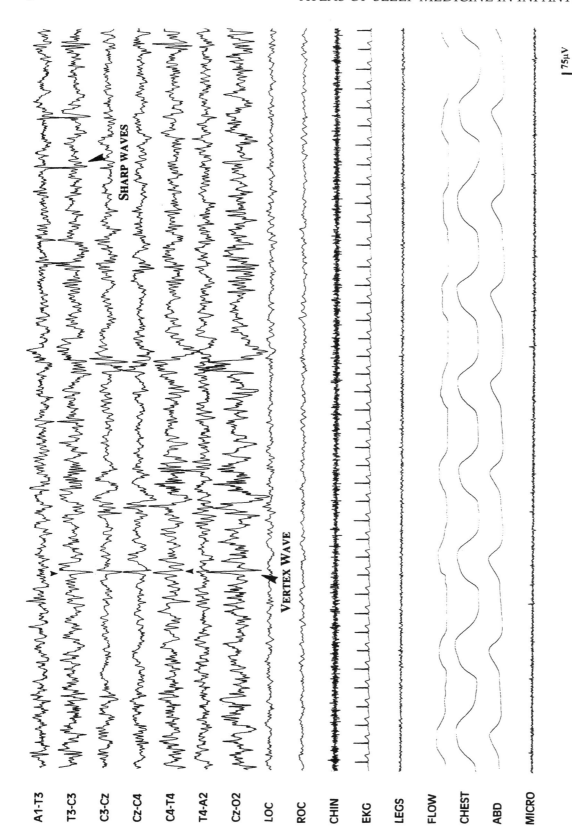

Digital Recording of Standard Pediatric Polysomnogram Montage

Figure 3. Digital Recording of Standard Pediatric Polysomnogram Montage

A bipolar EEG electrode array is demonstrated in this polysomnographic segment recorded from an 8-year-old male. Stage 2 sleep is demonstrated. This electrode array is especially useful in children and in differentiating vertex waves (V waves) from epileptiform activity. Note V waves originating from the vertex (small arrowhead) from epileptiform sharp waves originating from the left temporal region (large arrowhead).

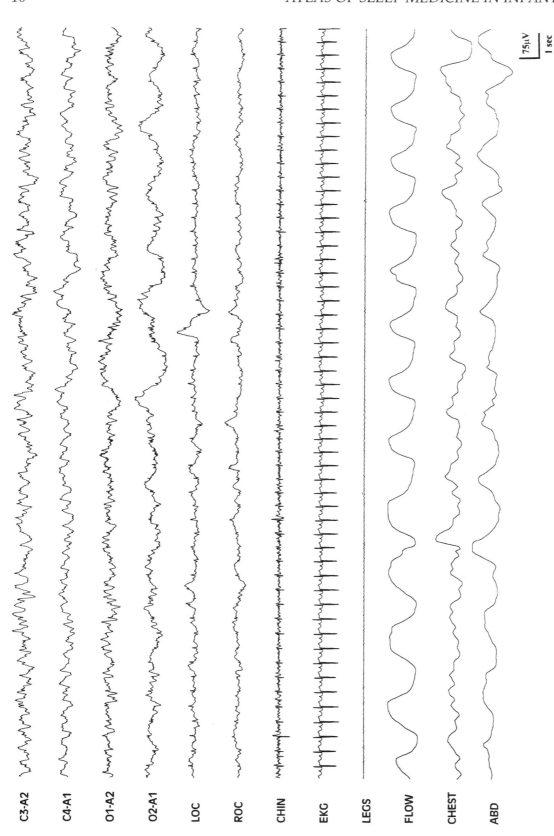

C3-A2

C4-A1

O1-A2

O2-A1

LOC

ROC

CHIN

EKG

LEGS

FLOW

CHEST

ABD

75μV
1 sec

Pediatric Polysomnogram Montage: Thermistry versus Capnography

Figure 4a. Pediatric Polysomnogram Montage: Thermistry versus Capnography

Figures 4a and 4b show polysomnographic segments recorded from a 4-year-old female who had a history of loud snoring associated with pauses and snorts. Tonsillar hypertrophy was noted on physical examination.

Although recording differential temperatures between inspired and expired air is reliable in adults, maintenance of the thermistor in the air stream is often difficult in children. Recording artifact is common. In addition, limited information is available from thermistry's qualitative signal. With partial obstruction of the upper airway, persistently elevated expired carbon dioxide, indicating alveolar hypoventilation, cannot be demonstrated. Even in the presence of significant sleep-disordered breathing, oxygen saturation may appear normal.

Figure 4a reveals a relatively normal appearing respiratory pattern. Airflow was recorded by thermistry, and respiratory effort was recorded by piezo crystal belts. Oxygen saturation was not directly depicted on this segment. No specific respiratory abnormalities appear to be present on this epoch.

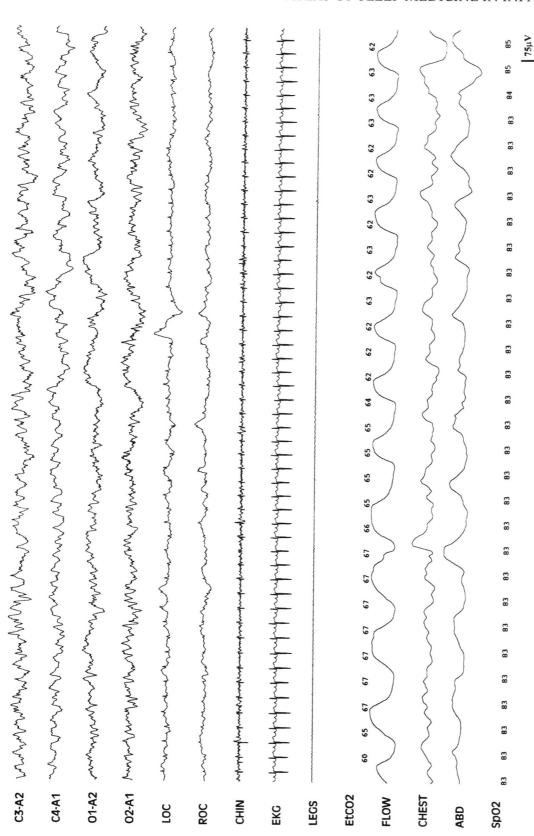

Pediatric Polysomnogram Montage: Thermistry versus Capnography

Figure 4b. Pediatric Polysomnogram Montage: Thermistry versus Capnography

Figure 4b is a depiction of a polysomnographic segment from the patient in Figure 4a, with side stream capnography and capnometry to record E_tCO_2. The ventilatory defect can now be clearly seen. Baseline oxygen saturation remains in the low 80s and E_tCO_2 is severely elevated.

When evaluating sleep-disordered breathing in children, it is recommended to record both airflow and E_tCO_2. Often, transcutaneous measurement of carbon dioxide is also helpful, especially when there is difficulty maintaining proper position of the cannula or when there is considerable ventilation of pulmonary dead space. Fluctuation in E_tCO_2 and elevated E_tCO_2 during recovery breaths after an apnea or hypopnea may be helpful in the assessment of sleep-disordered breathing in children.

Cannulae are placed in the nasal and oral air streams. Digital instrumentation presents several problems for visual analysis of the respiratory channels of polysomnographic segments. Because instrumentation requires aspiration of a minute quantity of air for sampling, there is a 3-second delay between graphic representation of effort and airflow. When there is skewing of airflow, brief central apneas may look very much like mixed apneas.

There is a 10-second delay in averaging of the E_tCO_2. Each numerical printout of E_tCO_2 represents the sampling average over the *prior* 10 seconds. During brief apneas, the capnometric average may only fall slightly despite a lowest E_tCO_2 of zero and highest of 60 mm Hg after recovery. Average E_tCO_2 would be 30 mm Hg over the 10 seconds of recording and would appear within the normal range.

A double-lumen nasal cannula is used in some patients, so that supplemental oxygen may be delivered while side stream E_tCO_2 is continuously measured.

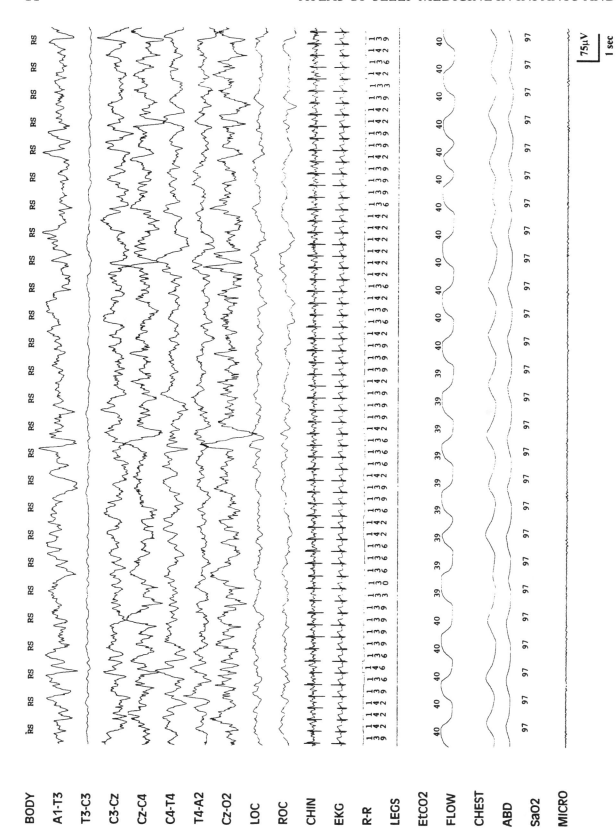

Standard Polysomnogram Montage: Double-Distance EEG Array

Figure 5a. Standard Polysomnogram Montage: Double-Distance EEG Array

Figure 5a represents a polysomnographic segment recorded from a 34-week-old premature infant weighing 1.5 kg. Recording of EEG in these very small patients requires careful scalp electrode placement, with electrodes far enough apart to minimize artifact.

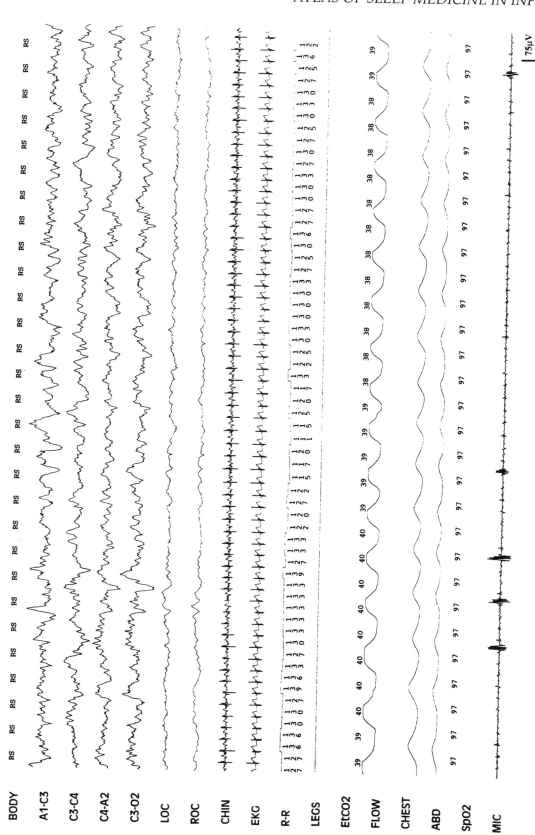

Standard Polysomnogram Montage: Double-Distance EEG Array, *continued*

Figure 5b. Standard Polysomnogram Montage: Double-Distance EEG Array

Because of the small size of a premature infant's head, a *salt bridge* between two electrodes can result, shorting out the electrical signal and rendering the EEG uninterpretable. Note the "flat line" artifact in channel T3-C3. This problem can be easily overcome by employment of a double-distance array in which intermediate electrode sites of the International 10–20 system of electrode placement are skipped. This EEG electrode array is demonstrated in the polysomnographic segment recorded from the same patient.

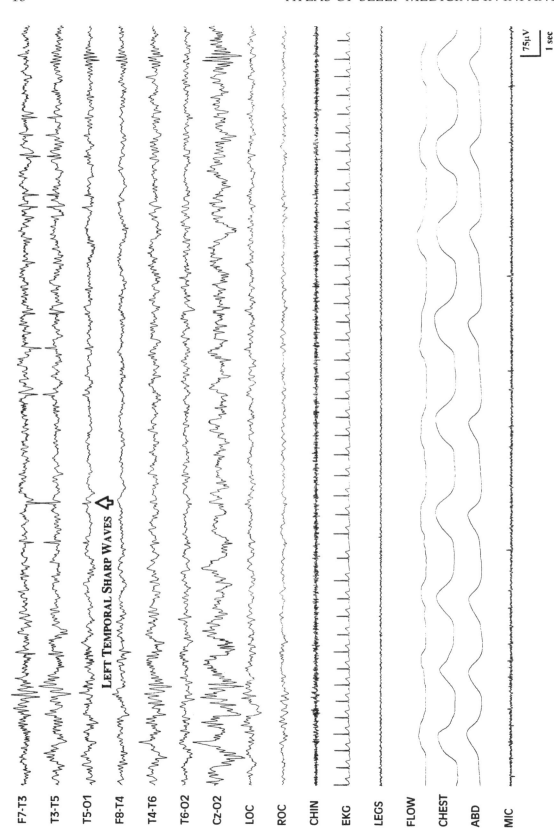

Bi-Temporal EEG Electrode Array

Figure 6. Bi-Temporal EEG Electrode Array

This polysomnographic segment was recorded from a 7-year-old male with a history of partial complex seizure disorder (absence seizures). This electrode array demonstrates the benefit of alternate EEG montage when evaluating children for seizures and some parasomnias. Temporal lobe seizures are not uncommon, and electrical epileptiform activity can often be more easily identified during sleep than wake. In this epoch, note frequent sharp wave activity located over the left temporal region. Epileptiform abnormalities may be seen in youngsters with temporal lobe seizures, but may also be suggestive of benign focal epilepsy of childhood, with centrotemporal spikes.

Although this limited electrode array cannot provide information that will be diagnostic of epilepsy, nor can it adequately identify the abnormal focus of activity, it can provide greater information than the standard polysomnographic referential montage typically used for recording adult polysomnograms.

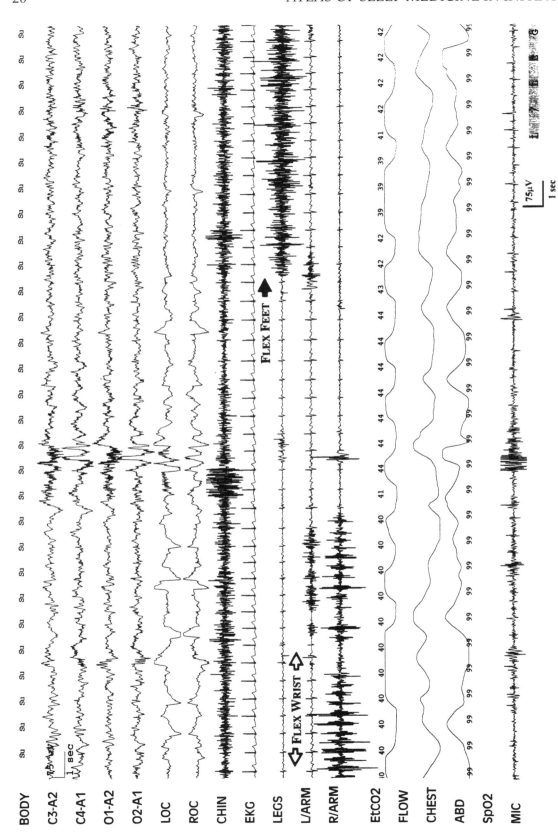

Montage for Assessing Periodic Limb Movement Disorder in Childhood

Figure 7. Montage for Assessing Periodic Limb Movement Disorder in Childhood

This polysomnographic epoch demonstrates a modified recording montage that may be used for detection of PLMS. This figure shows two central and two occipital standard referential EEG channels. Occipital EEG recordings are important for validation of arousals often associated with limb movements. EOG and Chin EMG provides the remaining channels needed for sleep stage scoring. EKG is lead 2. Note that both lower and upper limbs are being monitored. Bilaterally linked anterior tibialis EMG is supplemented with left and right wrist flexor muscle EMG. This montage, in combination with infrared video recording, provides for more precise polysomnographic assessment. The epoch displayed shows a portion of patient calibration recorded when the child was asked to flex his wrists and feet consecutively. Continuous EKG, capnography, capnometry, respiratory effort, and oxygen saturation are helpful for differentiating limb movements associated with arousals secondary to occult occlusive respiratory events associated with high upper airway resistance.

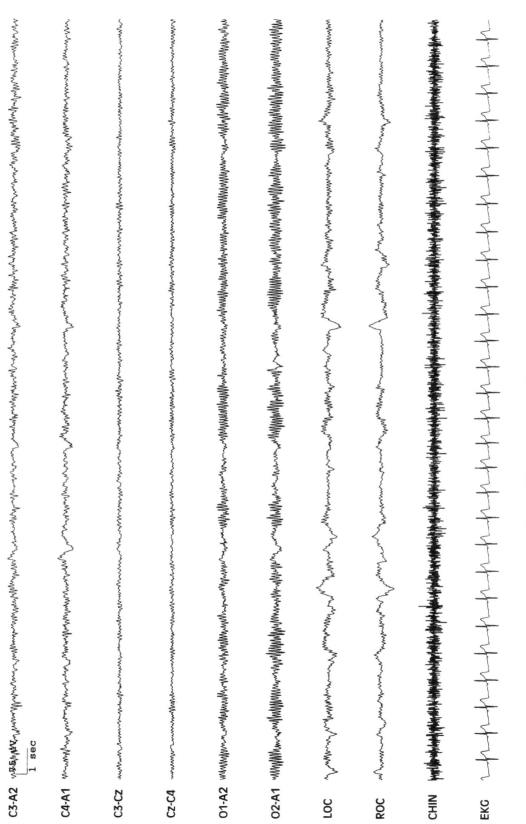

C3-A2

C4-A1

C3-Cz

Cz-C4

O1-A2

O2-A1

LOC

ROC

CHIN

EKG

Multiple Sleep Latency Test Montage

Figure 8a. Multiple Sleep Latency Test Montage

The polysomnographic segments in Figures 8a through 8c demonstrate a standard montage for recording the Multiple Sleep Latency Test (MSLT) in children. MSLT can provide objective evidence of daytime sleepiness and document the presence (or absence) of sleep onset REM periods (SOREMPs).

Each epoch displays two central EEG channels, two channels for recording occipital EEG activity, and two referential channels. Contralateral reference for both occipital recordings are used to maximize recording of alpha activity occurring during relaxed wakefulness with the eyes closed and to aid in observing the characteristic change to a mixed frequency EEG background seen at sleep onset. EOG and Chin EMG provide the remaining channels needed for sleep staging. This polysomnographic segment was recorded from an 8-year-old child during relaxed wakefulness with her eyes closed. Observe the rhythmic alpha EEG activity that is pervasive and maximal over the occiput.

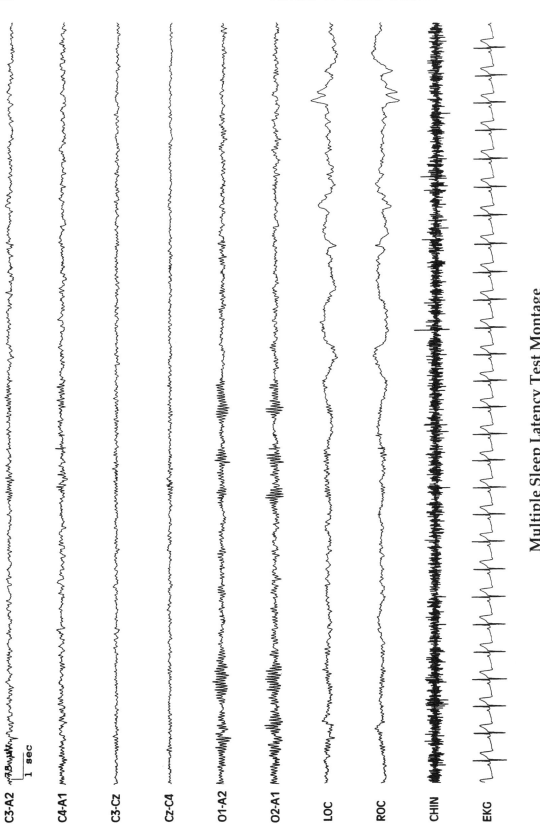

C3-A2

C4-A1

C3-Cz

Cz-C4

O1-A2

O2-A1

LOC

ROC

CHIN

EKG

75 µV
1 sec

Multiple Sleep Latency Test Montage

Figure 8b. Multiple Sleep Latency Test Montage

This figure demonstrates sleep onset. There is generalized EEG slowing and disappearance of the rhythmic alpha activity. Slow rolling eye movements are present.

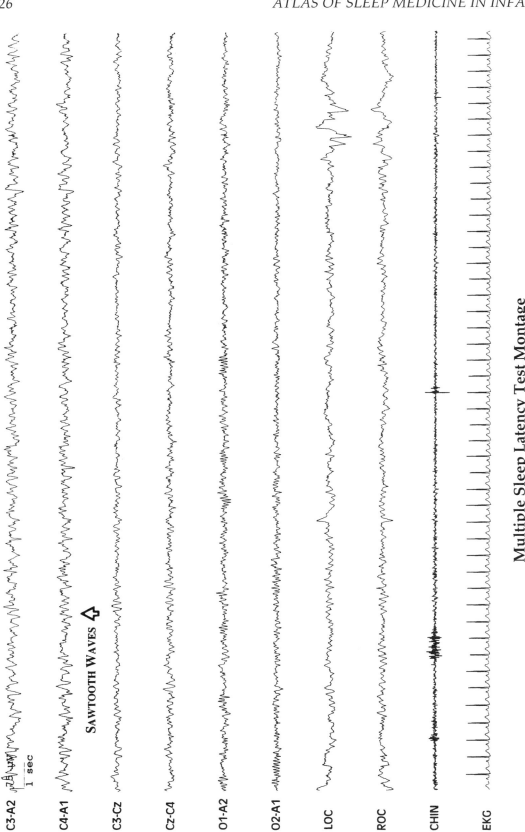

Multiple Sleep Latency Test Montage

Figure 8c. Multiple Sleep Latency Test Montage

This figure reveals the initial appearance of REM sleep. Sawtooth waves are maximal over the contralateral referenced central EEG lead placement (arrow).

Interpretation of MSLT is often difficult in children. Few normative data are available, especially in very young children. Assessment of MSLT data in youngsters is complex especially when daytime sleep is developmentally expected. Standard criteria can be modified, however, in order to attempt to assess degrees of daytime sleepiness in school-aged prepubertal, Tanner 1 children. Youngsters in this age range generally are quite alert throughout the day, and mean sleep onset latencies using adult criteria are typically considered normal. In our laboratory, three criteria are used to assess sleepiness. First, the mean sleep onset latency is *shorter than expected for age* in children with increased sleep pressure. Generally, a mean between 16 and 18 minutes is considered normal. If the mean sleep onset latency using five naps (and 20 minutes as the latency if sleep onset was not achieved: 'censored mean') is less than 16 minutes, sleepiness *might* be suspected. Second, because sleep onsets in a five-nap MSLT are unusual in youngsters during this developmental period, onset of sleep on three or more naps on a five-nap MSLT increases the suspicion of excessive daytime sleepiness. Finally, if sleep onset does not occur and/or sleep onset is considerably delayed, and there are *frequent microsleep periods* (epochs where polysomnographic sleep appears but is shorter than required to score a 30-second epoch as sleep), it again supports a presumption of excessive sleepiness.

None of the three criteria are diagnostic, nor are all three taken together diagnostic of excessive sleepiness. When taken in context of a child's history that supports the supposition of excessive daytime sleepiness, the diagnosis can be defended

Section II

Pneumography, Home Monitoring, and Event Recording

Pneumography is the recording of a limited number of physiological respiratory variables in an attempt to assess respiratory function. It has typically been performed in evaluation of apnea of prematurity and ALTEs.

As demonstrated in the following epochs and recording segments, many difficulties exist in the use of pneumography to assess sleep and sleep-related breathing disorders. First and most significant is poor sensitivity and specificity. Frequent false-positive and false-negative events are recorded. Impedance measurement of respiratory effort is quite inaccurate. For example, cardiac impulse is often detected as respiratory effort. State determination is also important in evaluation and assessment of a variety of respiratory patterns. Wakefulness and active sleep can be quite difficult to differentiate during unattended respiratory recordings. Since limited physiological parameters are recorded, obstructive apneas cannot be adequately characterized if they are not associated with significant gas exchange abnormalities. Often, occlusive respiratory events are brief (lasting at least two respiratory efforts without detection of airflow) and are associated with only minimal deceleration of heart rate. Prolonged central appearing pauses associated with "bradycardia" are often considered pathological. How-ever, many pauses can be normal physiological phenomena: for example, postsigh central apnea. In our laboratory, we have recorded postsigh respiratory pauses lasting up to 27 seconds.

Prolonged expiratory apnea may be associated with decreased instantaneous heart rate during the first third of the breathing pause. Instantaneous heart rate then returns to baseline as the pause continues. This variation in heart rate is similar to that seen during the Valsalva maneuver. In contrast, pathological central apneas are associated with heart rate deceleration as the apnea progresses, reaching its nadir during the last third of the respiratory pause. Clinical significance of expiratory apneas is unknown. Close analysis of raw data is required for differentiation of various types of normal and abnormal central appearing apneas.

Pneumograms are not screening tests, nor are they diagnostic investigations. Sensitivity is very poor. In addition, pneumograms are almost as expensive as comprehensive attended diagnostic polysomnography.

Suggested Reading

1. Consensus Statement: National Institutes of Health Development Conference on Infantile Apnea and Home

Monitoring, September 29–October 1, 1986. Pediatrics 1987;79:292–299.

2. Ferber R, Millman R, Coppola M, et al: Portable recording in the assessment of obstructive sleep apnea. ASDA standards of practice. Sleep 1994;17:378–392.

3. *Infantile Apnea and Home Monitoring.* U.S. Department of Health and Human Services, Public Health Service, National Institutes of Health, NIH Publication No. 87–2905, 1986.

4. *Report of the Michigan Ad Hoc Task Force on Apnea: A Consensus.* 2nd ed. Michigan Association of Apnea Professionals, 1992.

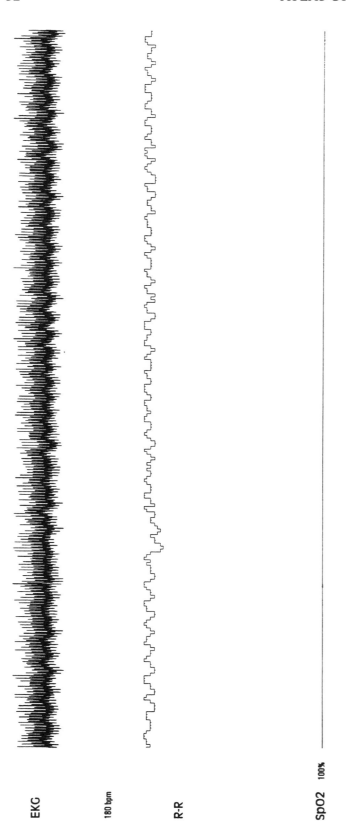

Pneumogram Recording from a 38-Week-Old Infant

EKG

180 bpm

R-R

SpO2   100%

IMPD

Figure 9a. Pneumogram Recording from a 38-Week-Old Infant

This figure represents a pneumogram segment recorded from a 38-week-old gestational-term infant who presented with a history of observed apnea at home. According to the infant's mother, the infant was pale and required vigorous stimulation to awaken and resume breathing. Unattended four-channel pneumography was done in the hospital's nursery.

Epoch length was 120 seconds, EKG and R-R interval were recorded, oxygen saturation was obtained by pulse oximetry, and respiratory effort by chest wall impedance. Sleep state was not recorded, nor can it be interpreted from this tracing. Respiration appears regular, heart rate is regular, and oxygen saturation is approximately 100%.

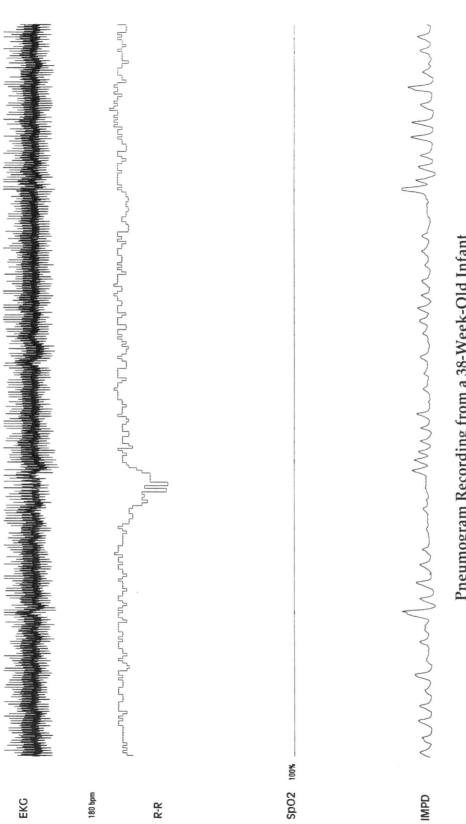

EKG

180 bpm

R-R

SpO2   100%

IMPD

Pneumogram Recording from a 38-Week-Old Infant

Figure 9b. Pneumogram Recording from a 38-Week-Old Infant

This pneumogram segment was recorded from the same infant as Figure 9a. There is an apparent fall in the heart rate, and chest wall impedance has decreased, suggesting a central apnea or hypopnea. Oxygen saturation has not changed, and S_pO_2 remains above 95%.

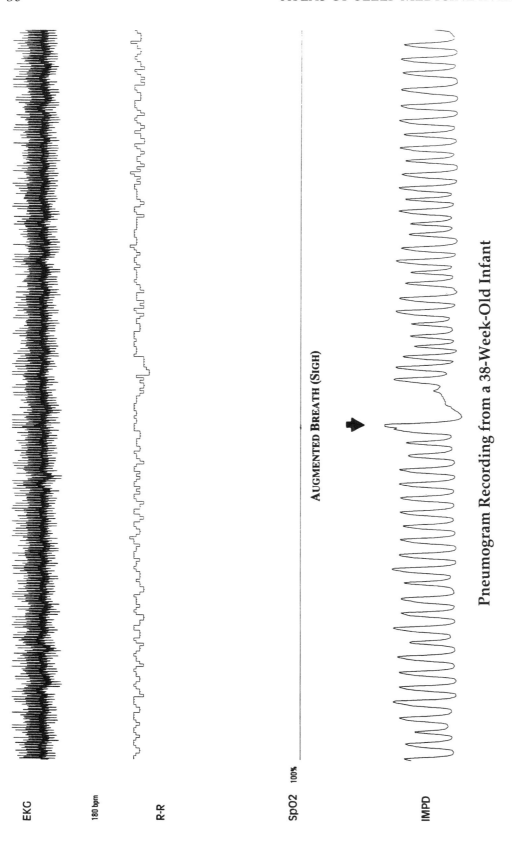

EKG

180 bpm

R-R

SpO2   100%

AUGMENTED BREATH (SIGH)

IMPD

Pneumogram Recording from a 38-Week-Old Infant

Figure 9c. Pneumogram Recording from a 38-Week-Old Infant

The pneumogram in Figure 9c reveals a 15-second respiratory pause following an augmented breath (sigh). Note that there is no change in heart rate or oxygen saturation despite the length of the respiratory pause (apnea).

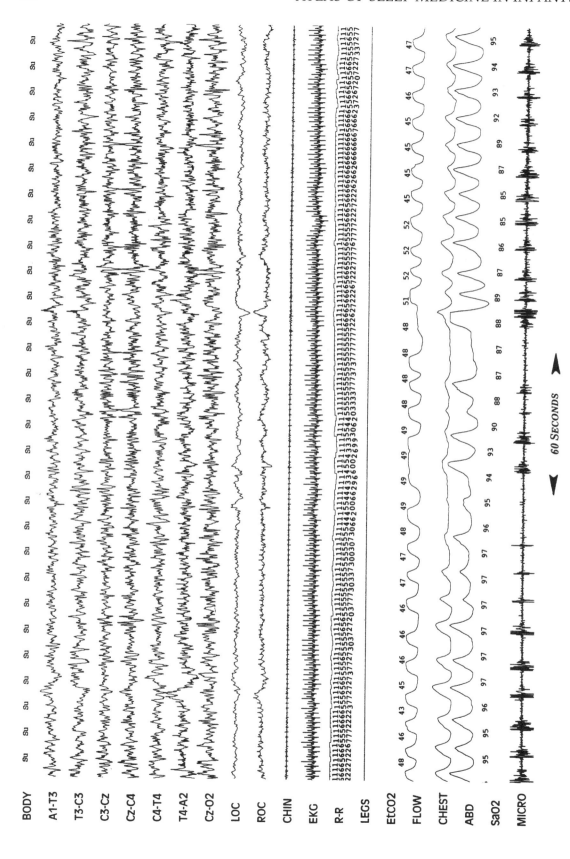

Polysomnographic Recording From a 38-Week-Old Infant

Figure 9d. Polysomnographic Recording From a 38-Week-Old Infant

This figure shows a 60-second segment of a comprehensive polysomnogram recorded from the same patient. The infant is in active sleep. Now the obstructive nature of this child's sleep-disordered breathing can be appreciated. Apneas are brief. Nonetheless, there is significant oxygen desaturation and increased E_tCO_2 during recovery breaths. Note that the infant reveals greater abdominal effort. Chest effort seems to decrease, suggesting increased diaphragmatic effort. If chest wall impedance was the only recording of respiratory effort, this event might have been misinterpreted as a central apnea.

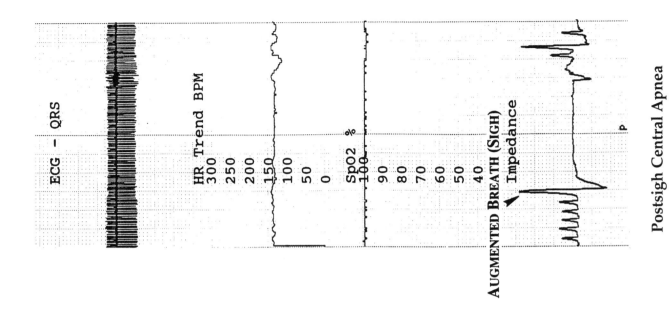

Postsigh Central Apnea

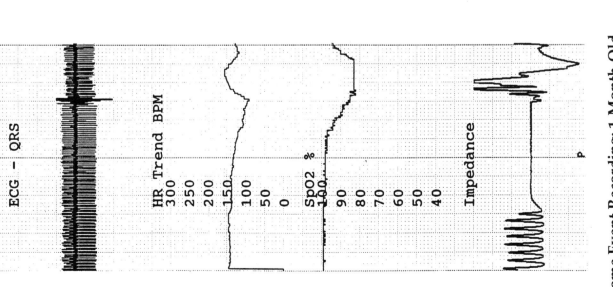

Home Event Recording; 1-Month-Old,
34-Week-Gestation Infant

Figure 10. Home Event Recording: 1-Month-Old, 34-Week-Gestation Infant

This event recording segment was recorded from a 1-month-old infant who was born at 34 weeks' gestation. She experienced an ALTE at home. Treatment included oral theophylline and continuous monitoring with a home apnea monitor. She was otherwise healthy and growing well. Past history and family history were unremarkable. Physical examination was normal and the child was neuro-developmentally appropriate for her corrected chronological age. Frequent apnea alarms were reported by parents.

In this segment, there is noticeable absence of impedance signal for more than 20 seconds on the depicted recorded event. Respiration appears regular for eight breaths prior to the pause, and irregular after the pause. This respiratory irregularity most likely indicates arousal after the event that precipitated the alarm. It may also be due to parental stimulation. There is considerable heart rate deceleration and oxygen desaturation present. Therefore, this event might represent a pathological central apnea associated with apnea of prematurity, and comprehensive evaluation is required.

Apnea of prematurity is thought to be due to immaturity of the central control of breathing. It is defined as cessation of respiration lasting 20 seconds or longer. It may also be diagnosed if there is excessive periodic breathing (especially during quiet sleep), or if an apnea lasts less than 20 seconds but is associated with significant heart rate deceleration, oxygen desaturation, or the appearance of neurological symptoms or signs. Apnea of prematurity often responds well to methylxanthines (theophylline or caffeine) and typically resolves spontaneously by conceptional term.

Home event recordings are not diagnostic procedures, but may be helpful in longitudinal management of children with sleep-disordered breathing. *Event recordings should not be used for diagnostic or screening purposes.* Their utility lies in the determination of validity of monitor alarms.

Figure 11. Postsigh Central Apnea

This event recording segment represents a postsigh central apnea, and is most likely a normal physiological respiratory event. Breathing appears regular for about five breaths prior to an augmented breath (sigh). This is followed by cessation of impedance signal for approximately 31 seconds. An irregular breathing pattern follows the respiratory pause, possibly representing a spontaneous arousal or parental stimulation after response to the apnea alarm.

In comparison to the prolonged central apnea presented in Figure 10, this respiratory pause is not associated with significant heart rate change, nor is it associated with oxygen desaturation, despite its length.

Postsigh central apneas can result in monitor alarms, due to prolonged absence of impedance signal. These events are most likely normal physiological respiratory pauses during sleep, perhaps related to the Herring-Breuer pulmonary stretch reflex. If these events are considered abnormal or pathological, prolonged use of apnea monitors may occur.

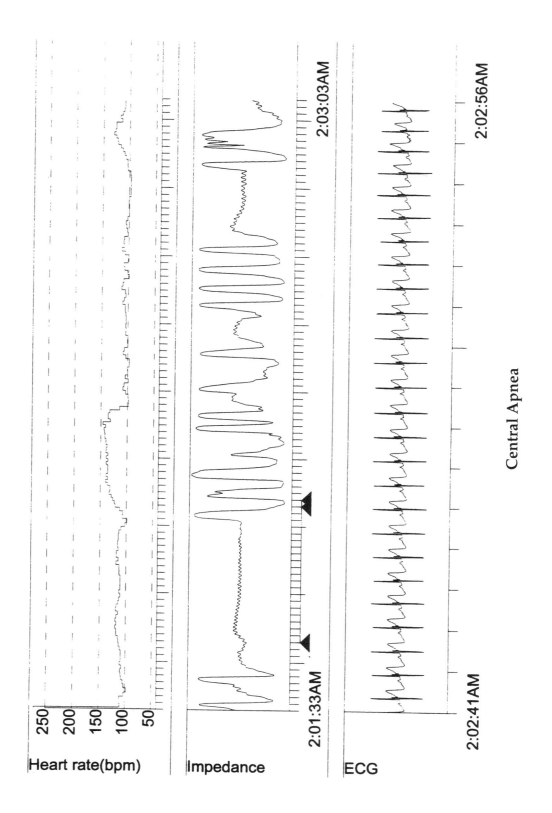

Central Apnea

Figure 12. Central Apnea

This event recording segment was obtained from a 6-month-old female who presented with a history of gastroesophageal reflux, sucking and swallowing abnormalities, and mild hypotonia. She was placed on an apnea monitor shortly after birth because of observed apneas that were not associated with cyanosis. In this event, two central appearing apneas are noted, the first lasting approximately 21 seconds and the second lasting about 12 seconds. There is respiratory variability present between the two apneas. Cardiac acceleration occurs after the first event. EKG reveals a sinus rhythm. Although S_pO_2 was not measured, parents responded to the alarm and noted no color change. From the event recording alone, however, it is impossible to determine sleep state. Similar recordings may occur during wakefulness.

Central apneas are normal physiological phenomena occurring most often during REM/active sleep. They are typically associated with other indications of normal respiratory instability of active sleep, and are not typically associated with significant oxygen desaturation or EKG deceleration.

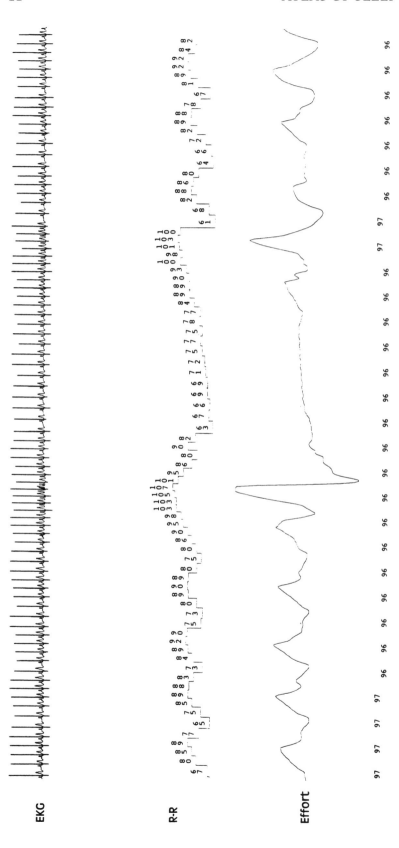

EKG

R-R

Effort

SpO2

Prolonged Expiratory Apnea

Figure 13. Prolonged Expiratory Apnea

This segment was recorded from a 3-year-old male who presented with a history of making unusual noises, grunting, and moaning during sleep. There was a history of loud snoring and restless sleep. An initial rise in the heart rate can be seen during an augmented breath immediately preceding the respiratory pause. Heart rate falls abruptly, reaches its nadir during the first third of the pause, and then gradually rises to baseline. Note normal oxygen saturation during and after the event. Compare this respiratory pause to the pathological central apnea presented in Figure 10, in which there is progressive deceleration of heart rate and oxygen saturation during the apnea. Both instantaneous heart rate and oxygen saturation reach nadirs during the latter portion of the pathological apnea. Clinical significance of prolonged expiratory apnea is unclear at present.

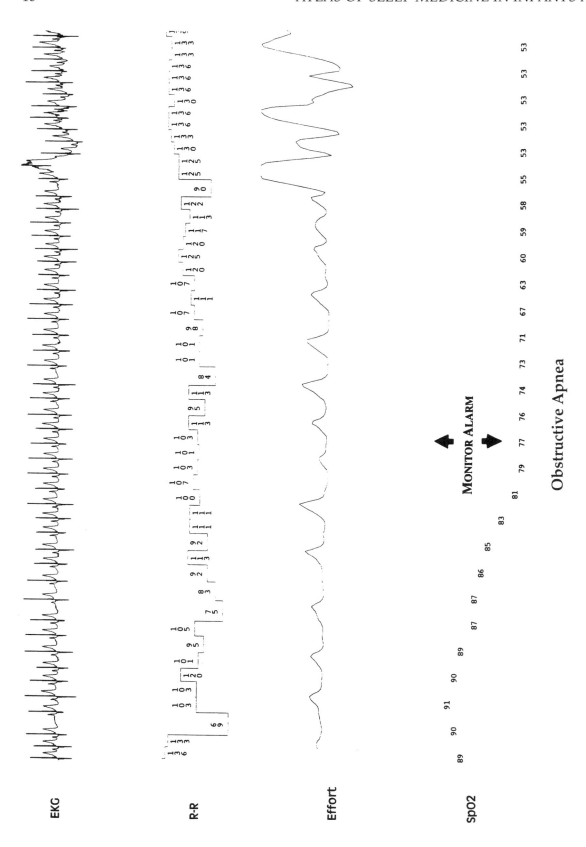

Figure 14. Obstructive Apnea

This segment was recorded from an 8-month-old male who presented with a history of frequent nocturnal awakenings. Behavioral interventions, despite adequate parental compliance, did not result in improvement of symptoms. Loud snoring was associated with pauses and snorts. Restless sleep and sleep-related diaphoresis was also described by his parents.

Respiratory effort is present in the impedance channel. Since these waveforms are not coincident with the EKG signal, pulse artifact is an unlikely cause for the graphic representation. There is fall in the instantaneous heart rate to a low of about 65 beats per minute. Oxygen saturation falls to a low of 52%. The child's monitor alarmed due to low oxygen saturation. Parents observed that the baby was breathing but somewhat dusky in color.

This event could be consistent with an obstructive apnea, and full polysomnographic analysis is required for accurate assessment. If oxygen saturation had not been monitored, this event may not have been identified as abnormal on either a limited channel pneumogram or event recording.

Obstructive sleep apneas cannot be adequately diagnosed or assessed by limited pneumography or by event recordings. Since nasal/oral airflow is typically not continuously monitored with these procedures, only two physiological parameters may provide clues or suggest the presence of obstructive upper airway disorder: cardiac deceleration and oxygen desaturation in the presence of continued respiratory efforts.

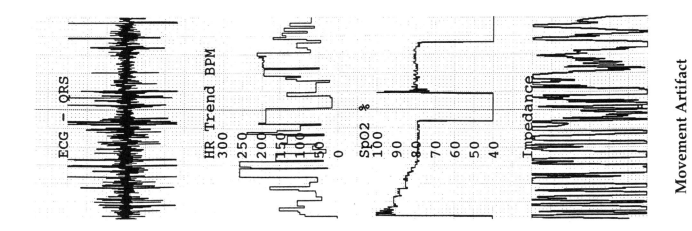

Movement Artifact

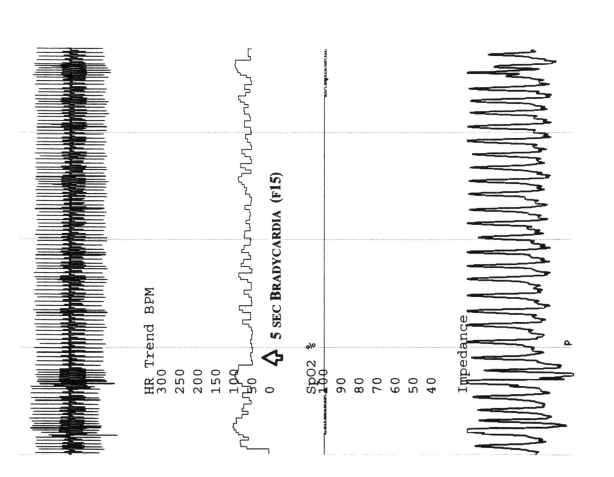

Sinus Bradycardia

Figure 15. Sinus Bradycardia

This event recording segment was obtained from a 14-month-old toddler who had been monitored for approximately 1 year after experiencing an ALTE. Initially, parents reported frequent apnea alarms. Mother and father took turns sleeping on the floor in the child's room in order to rapidly respond to the alarms. After 7 months of age, apnea alarms became rare, but monitor alarms for bradycardia remained frequent. The segment identified by the arrow is the 5 seconds of heart rate less than 60 beats per minute required for the monitor to alarm. Cardiotachometry and QRS recording suggested sinus rhythm at an average rate of about 64 beats per minute. This was confirmed by prolonged continuous EKG (Holter) monitoring. Note that there is no change in oxygen saturation, nor is there change in respiratory pattern. Lowest instantaneous heart rate was approximately 47 beats per minute.

Although cardiac deceleration can occur during obstructive and central apneas, low heart rate alarms may frequently occur because the monitor threshold for alarm is set too high for the patient's developmental age.

Figure 16. Movement Artifact

This event recording segment was obtained from a 5-month-old infant who was born at 35 weeks' gestation. He was noticed to experience several apneas in the nursery, caffeine was prescribed, and he was discharged to home on an apnea monitor. Monitor alarms occurred approximately 4 to 6 times per night. Parents responded quickly to the alarms, but after each alarm, the infant was found to be breathing normally, color was normal, and there was a normal heart rate.

Note the extreme irregularity and movement artifact in all channels. Irregularity of respiratory rate and apparent movement have resulted in this recording artifact. The monitor detected it as a low heart rate of 16 beats per minute. Visual analysis of raw data from each event recording epoch is required in order to accurately rule out artifact as the cause of alarms.

Section III

Recording Artifacts

Recording artifacts, in even the best run polysomnogram, are inevitable. Artifacts may be related to the patient, the equipment, or the recording environment. Attended studies are mandatory because movement and tactile defensiveness of young children often results in displacement of sensors and leads.

Most recording artifacts are transient, but some may become continuous and may obscure the record enough to render it uninterpretable. Recognizing artifacts, documenting the artifact on the recording, and *fixing the problem* require technical expertise and vigilance. *The most important variable in obtaining a reliable and reproducible polysomnogram with minimal interference is the technician.*

Some patient-generated artifacts are caused by sweating, touching or pulling the electrodes, movement and muscle activity, sucking, and chewing. Sometimes older children will create voluntary artifact.

The most common environmental artifact is 60 Hz interference, which can be created by any electrical equipment within the recording environment. Other environmental artifacts can be mistaken for physiological events, eg, environmental noise causing frequent arousals, and ventilation of dead space resulting in a relatively low E_tCO_2. It is essential that the technician *closely monitor* the recording and document any and all interference that might decrease the quality of recording and the accuracy of interpretation. As long as artifact is appropriately identified, documented, and minimized, most pediatric polysomnograms can be adequately interpreted.

In very young patients and patients who cannot follow instructions, patient biocalibrations cannot be done. If a specific artifact is identified in the course of a recording, it may be recommended that the technician not disturb the child in order to eliminate certain artifacts or replace electrodes. It may be easier to wait for SWS to appear. At that time, the arousal threshold is quite high and repair of electrodes and patient sensors may be easily accomplished.

Suggested Reading

1. Cooper R, Osselton JW, Shaw JC: *EEG Technology.* 3rd ed. London: Butterworths & Company, 1980.
2. Cross C: Technical tips: Patient specific electrode application techniques. Am J EEG Technol 1992;32:86–92.
3. Daly DD, Pedley TA: *Current Practice of Clinical EEG.* 2nd ed. New York: Raven Press, 1990.
4. Gordon M: Artifacts created by imbalanced electrode impedance. Am J EEG Technol 1980;20:149–160.
5. Guilleminault C: *Sleeping and Waking Disorders, Indications and Techniques.* Menlo Park, CA: Addison-Wesley, 1982.
6. Picton TW, Hilliard SA: Cephalic skin potentials in electroencephalography. Electroencephalogr Clin Neurophysiol 1972;33:419–424.
7. Tyner F, Knott JR, Mayer WB: *Fundamentals of EEG Technology. Volume 1—Basic Concepts and Methods.* New York: Raven Press, 1983.

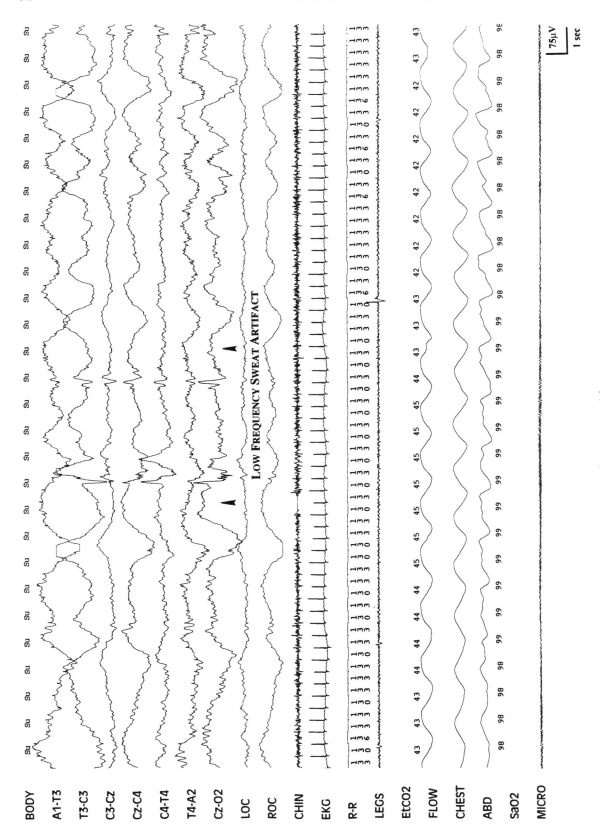

Sweat Artifact

Figure 17. Sweat Artifact

This polysomnographic segment was recorded from a 1-week-old infant. Acquisition was obtained by attended portable polysomnography in the pediatric intensive care unit isolation room. The 30-second epoch demonstrates low frequency sweat artifact in the EEG and EOG channels during quiet sleep. Frequency of these slow waves is much slower than respiration, eliminating respiratory movement artifact as a cause.

Electrolyte content of sweat modifies the composition of electro-conductive material. This modification and electrical potentials generated by sweat gland activity are thought to underlie the low fre-quency (usually 0.5 Hz or less) baseline oscillation. At times, this slow drift may be mistaken for slow waves, since the amplitude is often greater than 75 μV.

Sweat artifact can be symmetrical or asymmetrical. Note the asymmetry seen over the left temporal EEG recording. Sweating may be secondary to environmental conditions or may be endogenous. In the laboratory it is often created by warm environmental temperatures, sleep-related diaphoresis (eg, diaphoresis associated with obstructive sleep apnea), or wrapping the child's head in order to protect the electrodes. The best method to eliminate sweat artifact is to cool the patient and/or reapply the electrodes.

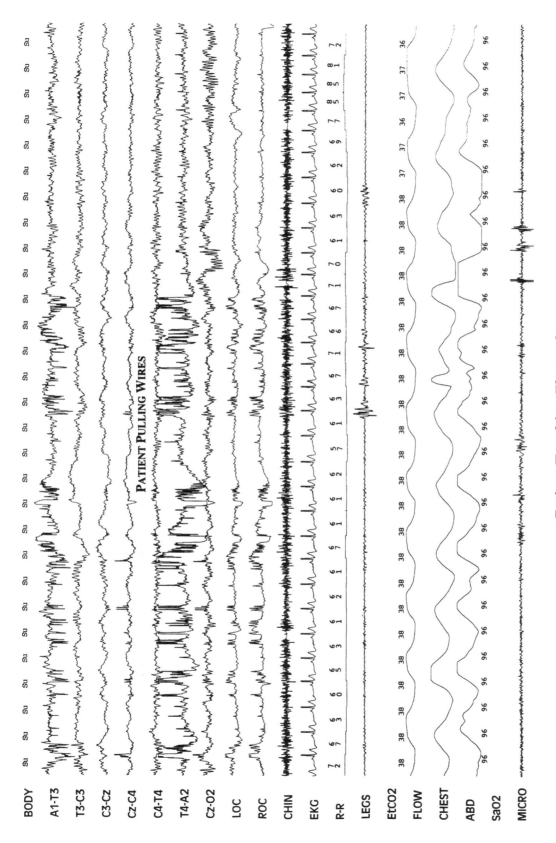

Figure 18. Patient Touching Electrodes

This figure is a polysomnographic segment recorded from an 8-year-old child who, while undergoing an in-patient psychiatric evaluation, had been noted to snore loudly during sleep. He did not tolerate attachment of the scalp electrodes with collodion. Electrodes were held in place by an elasticized bandage placed over the electrodes and gently wrapped around the child's head. Artifact Significant subject-based artifact is seen during this tracing. Artifact

was produced by the youngster pulling on a group of bundled EEG and EOG electrode lead wires. Abrupt vertical transients were documented with each "tug" on the lead bundle, but were not seen over all recording channels. This artifact was a result of sudden changes in electrode impedance as each electrode was pulled from direct contact with the scalp. It was corrected by imbedding each electrode cup in a larger portion of electroconductive material. Care must be taken, however, to avoid creating a salt bridge between electrode cups.

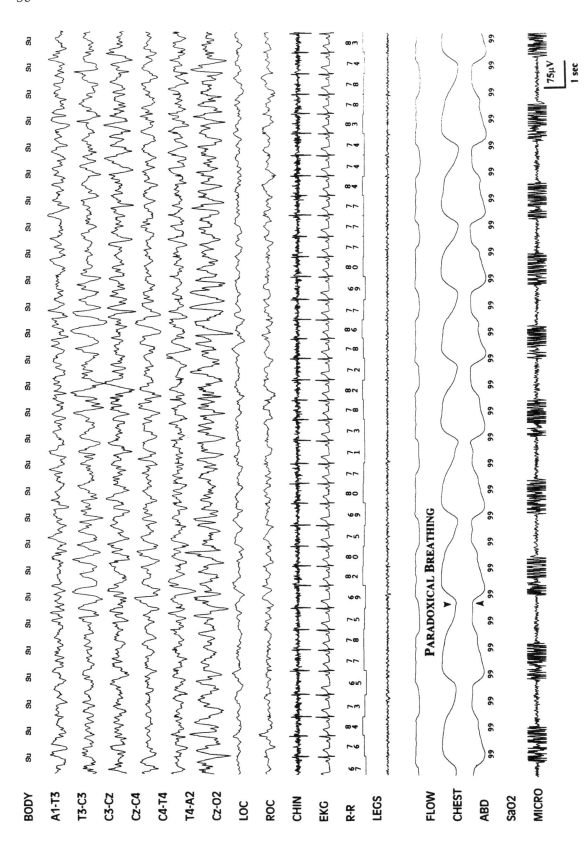

Poor Airflow Recordings

Figure 19a. Poor Airflow Recordings

The polysomnographic segment in this figure was obtained from a 10-year-old male with a history of loud snoring associated with pauses and snorts, restless sleep, and excessive daytime sleepiness. Airflow was recorded by thermistry. There is poor oscillation of the flow recording due to displacement of the nasal/oral thermistor used to derive the signal. The patient was supine, but he had his thumb in his mouth and his hand interfered with proper placement in the air stream. Both nasal and oral portions of the thermistor were found to be bent. Chest and abdominal respiratory efforts are 180° out of phase and snoring is recorded sonographically.

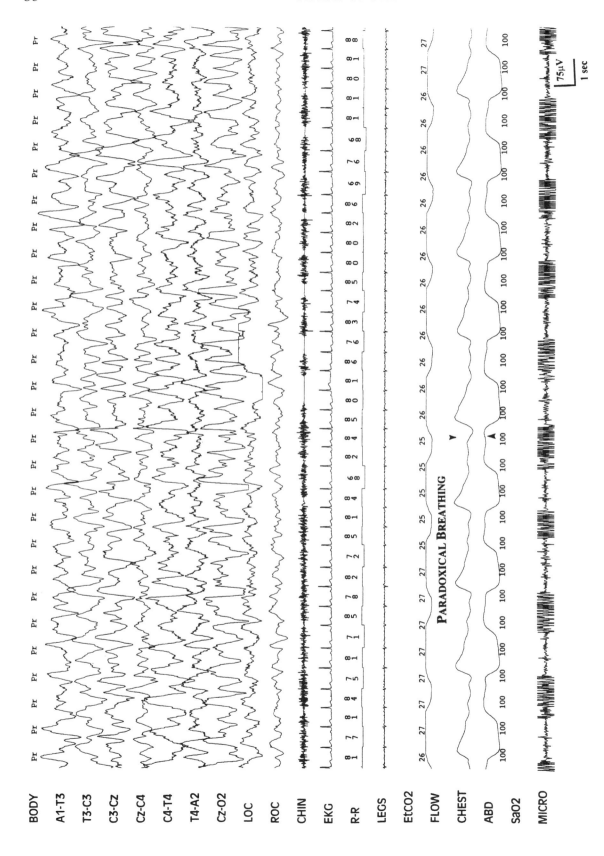

Poor Airflow Recordings

Figure 19b. Poor Airflow Recordings

This figure shows a recording taken during SWS from an 8-year-old female being studied for sleep-disordered breathing. History was significant for loud snoring, restless sleep, and enuresis. Adeno-tonsillar hypertrophy was noted. Airflow was recorded using capnography. Poor flow recording was due to displacement of the nasal/oral cannula from the air streams. Capnometry average is low due to mixing of expired air with room air. When the cannula was repositioned, capnometry average was 52 mm Hg and remained above 50 mm Hg for the remainder of the recording, indicating obstructive hypoventilation. Chest and abdominal effort recordings are 180° out of phase and snoring is recorded sonographically.

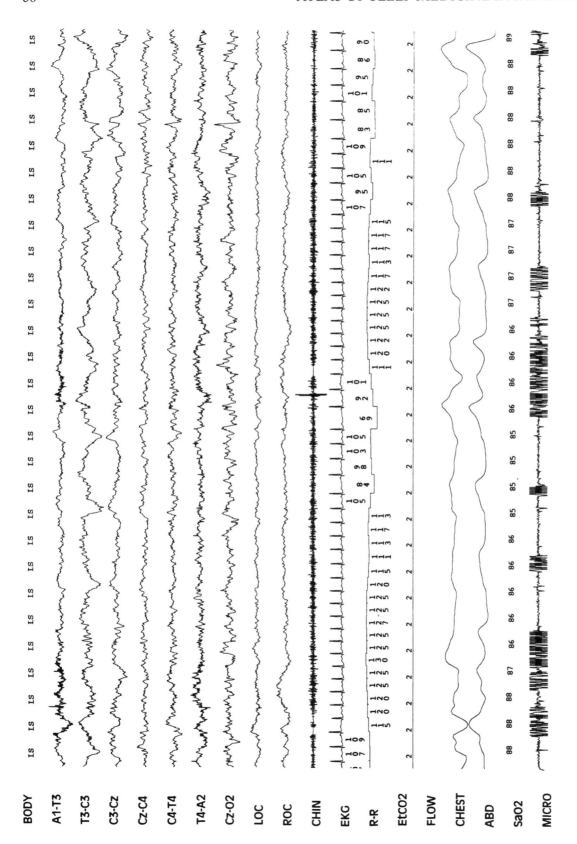

Poor Airflow Recordings

Figure 19c. Poor Airflow Recordings

This polysomnographic segment was recorded during stage 1 sleep from a 2-year-old female with a history of restless sleep, chronic sinusitis, and reactive airways disease. Profuse nasal discharge was present during the night of the study. This polysomnographic segment demonstrates occlusion of the cannula used to derive the capnographic signal. No airflow is apparent. Despite the absence of airflow signal, note the augmented respiratory efforts, loud snoring, and oxygen desaturation observed at the termination of what appear to be hypopneic events. This recording artifact is corrected by changing the cannula and the water trap on the capnometer.

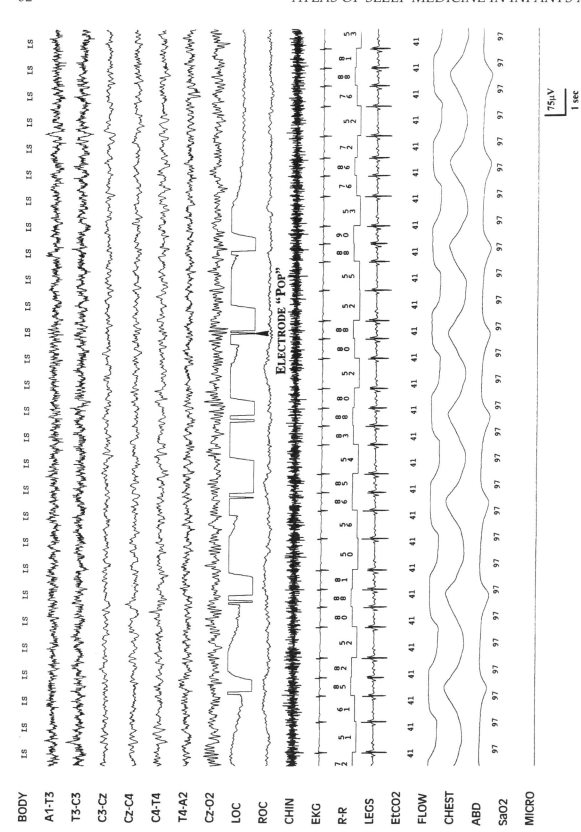

Electrode Pops

Figure 20. Electrode Pops

This polysomnographic segment was recorded from a 6-year-old female who was being evaluated in the sleep lab after suffering a significant injury during an episode of agitated sleep walking. Electrode "pop" artifact is present in the left EOG channel (LOC). Sudden change in electrode impedance by partial loss of contact with the skin surface results in an abrupt shift in the recording. In this epoch, representation of electrode pop artifact is not transient, but is associated with respiratory effort. Artifact starts during the inspiratory phase of each respiratory cycle. The child is lying on her left side, and is likely lying on the electrode.

Electrode pops are common artifacts encountered during polysomnography. They can be seen in any electrode array. Pops seem to be due to an abrupt change in electrode impedance caused either by poor electrode attachment resulting in partial loss of contact with the skin surface, insufficient electroconductive material, drying of the electroconductive material, or a combination of factors.

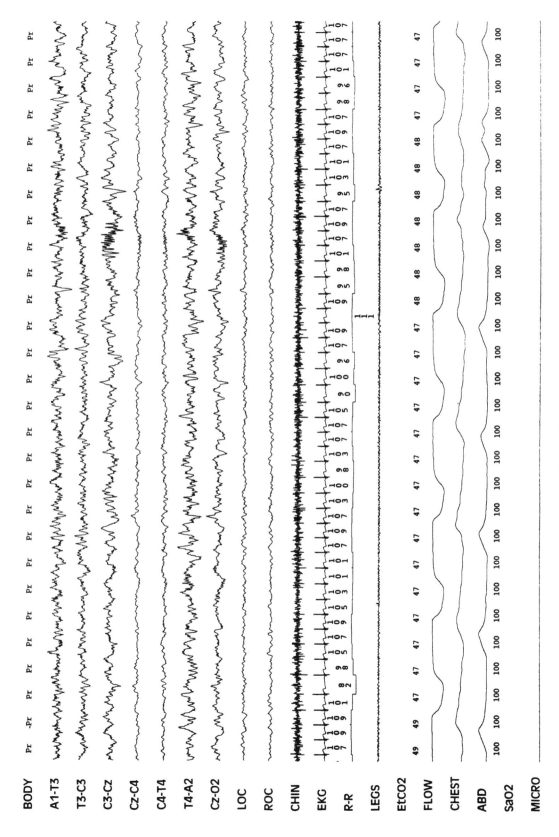

Broken Electrode Wire

Figure 21. Broken Electrode Wire

This polysomnographic epoch was recorded from a 3-year-old female patient. During the course of the recording, the child demonstrated extreme tactile defensiveness and pulled on the EEG bundle. The wire attached to the C4 electrode cup was inadvertently separated from the cup, but still made contact with the electrode. Continuous 60 Hz interference was noted by the technician. The 60 Hz filter was engaged and the sensitivity lowered, resulting in the recording above. Electrode impedance was checked and found to be greater than 5000 Ω in the Cz-C4 and C4-T4 channels. C4 was identified as the common electrode and the source of the artifact. The damaged electrode was replaced and the recording resumed. If the 60 Hz filters had been initially engaged and impedance not checked, artifact might have been filtered from the recording and the interpreter may not have questioned contamination.

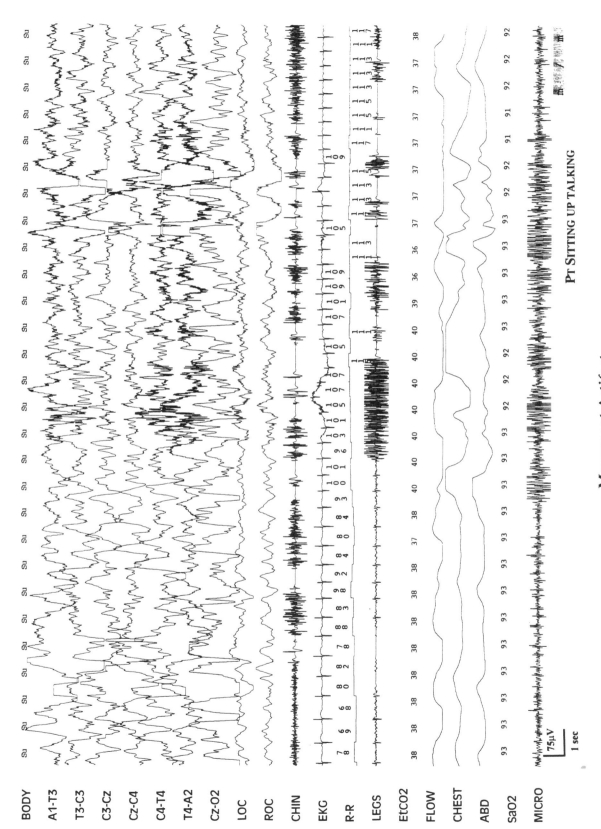

Movement Artifact

Figure 22. Movement Artifact

This polysomnographic segment was recorded from a 3-year-old male who was suffering from severe sleep terrors. Spells were occurring nightly and, on occasion, several times per night. This segment displays movement artifact, which can be seen throughout most of the channels. These movements represent the initial portion of a partial arousal. Movement was associated with the youngster sitting up in bed and vocalizing, which was both seen on video recording and documented directly on the record by the technician.

Superimposed muscle activity can be seen over the central and temporal areas of the EEG. Artifactual slow frequency deltalike waves due to electrode and wire movement can also be seen over most of the EEG and EOG signals. Increased submental and anterior tibialis EMG with movement-associated blocking is demonstrated, as is movement artifact obscuring the EKG recording. Note the erratic airflow and respiratory effort recorded during the major body movements as well as the representation of vocalizations recorded on the sonogram.

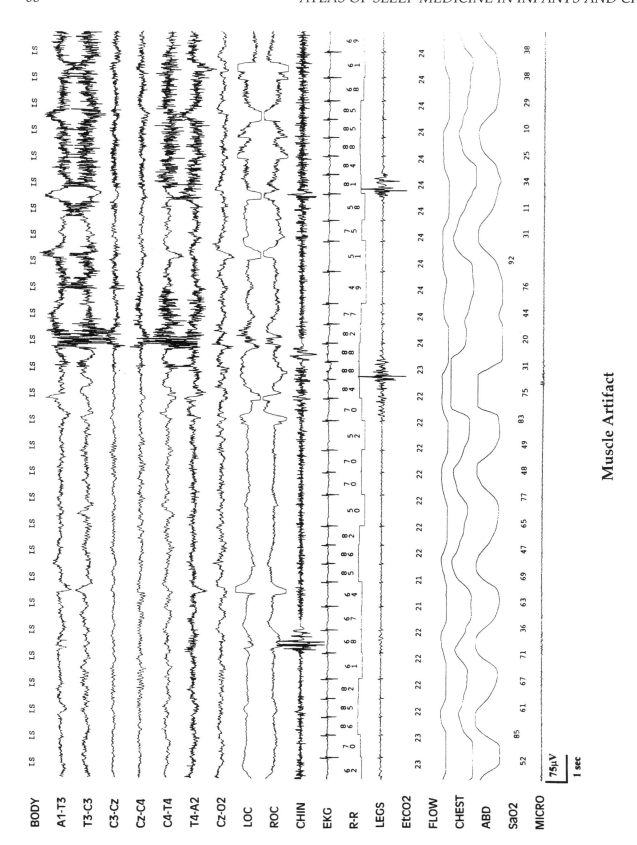

Muscle Artifact

Figure 23. Muscle Artifact

This polysomnographic epoch was recorded during a period of prolonged wakefulness after sleep onset in a 5-year-old female being studied for possible obstructive sleep apnea. Muscle artifact is superimposed over the EEG channels. Artifact was greatest in the central and temporal regions bilaterally. This muscle artifact was produced by the child's stern facial expression and clenched teeth. Note the superimposed fast activity, which completely obscures the recording.

Superimposition of muscle artifact is common during pediatric polysomnography. Gross body movements frequently occur and cover the recording. Technician documentation is quite important because interpretation of movements during wakefulness and during sleep may not be clear from the recording alone.

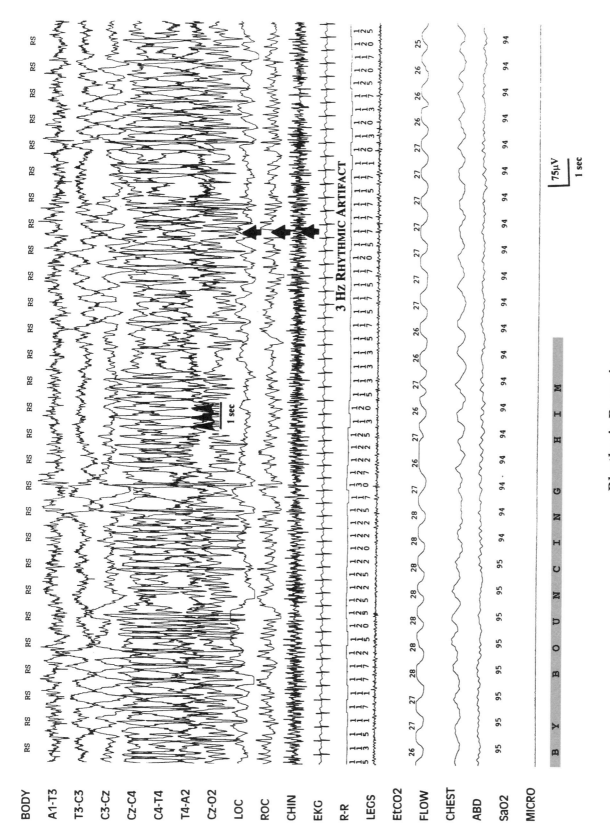

Rhythmic Bouncing

Figure 24. Rhythmic Bouncing

This polysomnographic segment was recorded from a 4-month-old male who had suffered an ALTE at home and was undergoing polysomnography as part of a comprehensive assessment. The infant was having difficulty settling in the laboratory, and his father attempted to soothe him by bouncing him on his knee. Rhythmic high voltage artifact occurs at a frequency of approximately 3 Hz and is concentrated over the right hemisphere. Note the baby's body position is right side.

Abrupt repetitive movements can be seen in children with rhythmic movement disorders, but this artifact typically occurs at a slower frequency. In this epoch, relatively fast frequency movement artifact can be seen superimposed over EEG, EOG, EMG, and effort signals. This is a common artifact seen in infant polysomnograms when parents try to soothe the child. When documented correctly, it is easily distinguishable from biological signals. It is caused by movement of electrodes during the rhythmic activity.

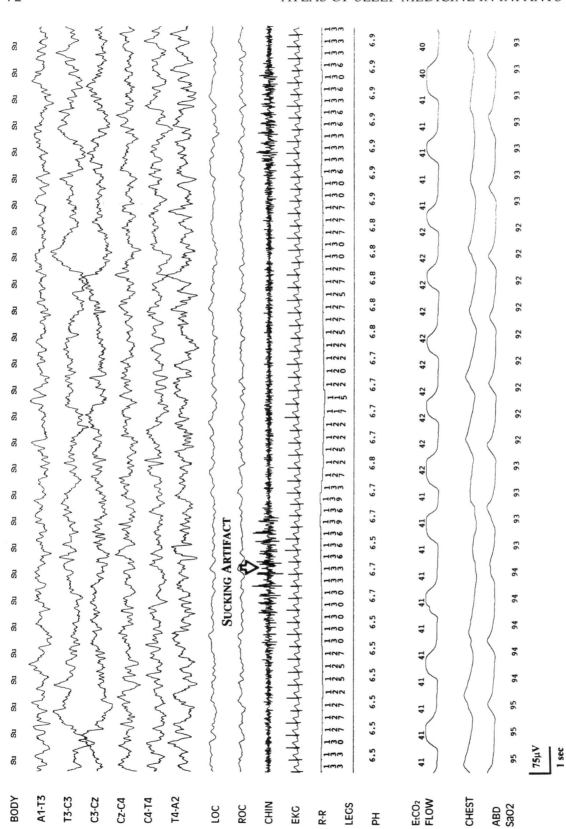

Sucking Artifact

Figure 25. Sucking Artifact

This polysomnographic segment was recorded from a 1-month-old male, and demonstrates sucking artifact seen on the submental EMG channel. This artifact is recorded as waxing and waning of the chin EMG tone lasting about 5 seconds, and occurs as a result of submental muscle activity during sucking and swallowing. Sucking behavior is usually seen on polysomnography in infants and young children. Neonates and young infants may exhibit this behavior spontaneously. Older infants and young children manifest this artifact when sucking on a pacifier, bottle, or finger. It may begin during wakefulness and continue during quiet sleep. Phasic activity is noted during active sleep and may involve intermittent chin muscle movements. The artifact observed on this epoch was produced due to the infant sucking on a pacifier.

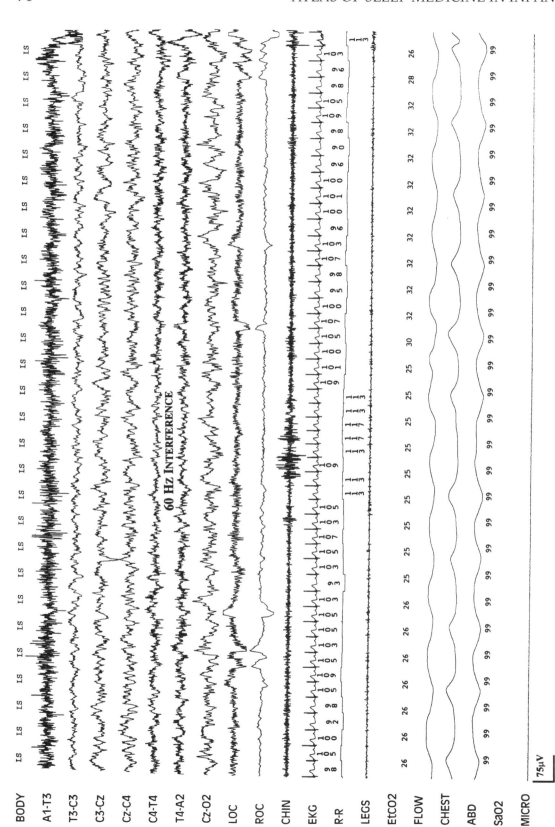

60 Hz Interference

Figure 26. 60 Hz Interference

This polysomnographic segment was recorded from a 10-year-old male who was being evaluated for sleep-disordered breathing. The epoch was obtained immediately after patient set-up and prior to performance of patient calibrations. Channels A1-T3 and LOC display 60 Hz interference. This is the most common environmental artifact encountered during polysomnography. It may be a result of any electromagnetic equipment in the immediate vicinity of the recording equipment. However, 60 Hz interference can also be caused by poor electrode-scalp interface and/or drying of the electroconductive material used between the electrode cup and skin.

Interference of 60 Hz may be blocked by the filter; however, recording equipment should be shielded from this type of environmental artifact. When it does occur, electrode impedance should be checked. In the epoch demonstrated, impedance was greater than 5000 Ω in the A1 lead. A1, as the common electrode in both derivations, was removed and reapplied, and the artifact subsequently resolved.

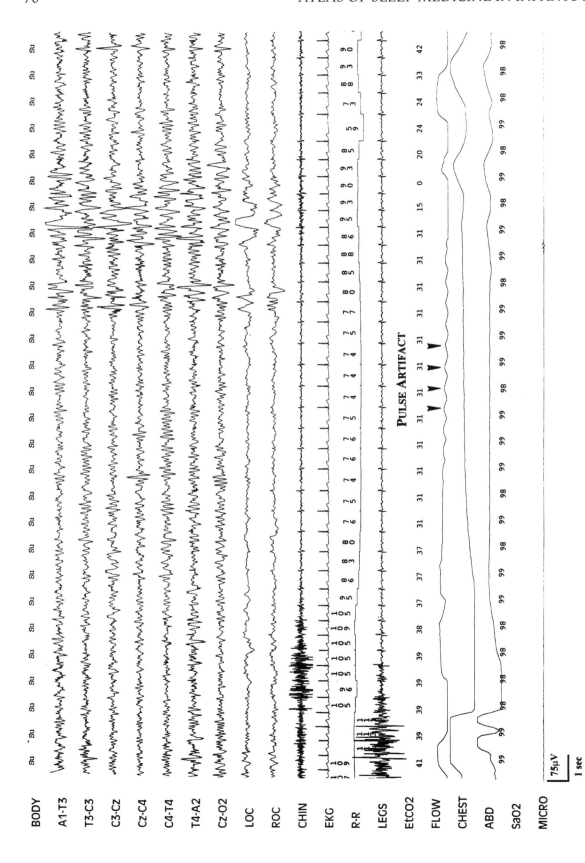

Pulse Artifact

Figure 27. Pulse Artifact

This polysomnogram segment was recorded from a 3-year-old female being studied because of prolonged respiratory pauses that occurred during sleep. Based on pneumographic recording, these pauses had previously been interpreted as pathological central apneas. Pulse artifact can be seen in the flow channel. There are negative deflections of the tracing seen, that are not associated with respiratory effort and are not occurring at the same rate as respiration. Each deflection corresponds with the heart rate, and each appears to be occurring during the diastolic phase of the cardiac cycle. Pulse artifact is thought to be due to expression of small amounts of air from lung dead space when the heart pushes outward during diastole. In thin individuals, pulse artifact from aortic pulsation can also be seen in the effort channels.

A second form of pulse artifact exists and typically occurs in the EEG channels. There is regular deflection of the tracing in conjunction with arterial pulsation. It occurs when an electrode is placed directly over a scalp artery, and there is movement of the electrode with each pulsation.

Although the displayed respiratory pause shown in this figure lasts for approximately 21 seconds, there are several characteristics that distinguish it from a pathological central apnea. First, there is a preceding arousal and augmented breath (sigh). Second, heart rate fall occurs early in the event, with rise of the instantaneous heart rate to baseline as the respiratory pause continues. Finally, there is no significant variation in oxygen saturation, despite the prolonged nature of cessation of respiration.

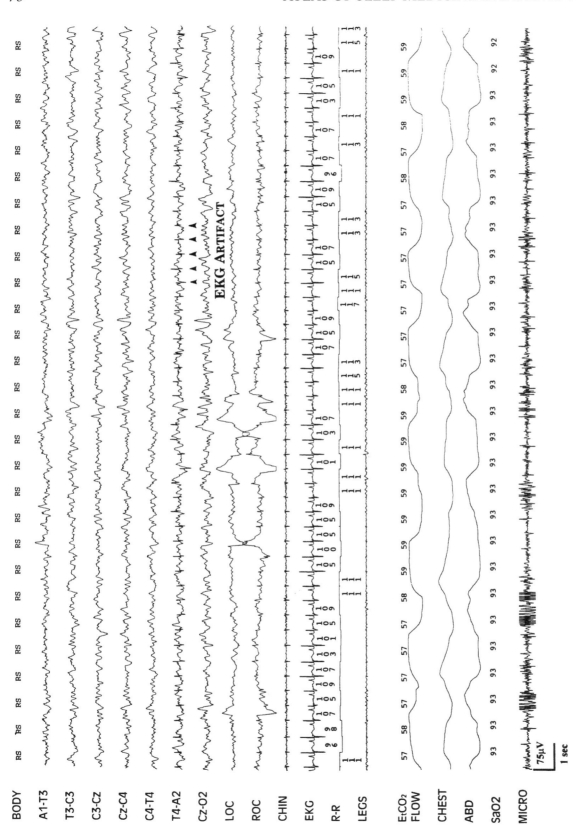

EKG Artifact

Figure 28. EKG Artifact

This polysomnogram segment was recorded from a 6-year-old male with a history of loud snoring associated with pauses and snorts. There was also a complaint of extreme hyperactivity alternating with periods of excessive somnolence. He was having considerable difficulty paying attention in school. This 30-second epoch recorded during REM sleep demonstrates very significant obstructive hypoventilation. EKG artifact is present in T4-A2 and in the chin muscle EMG.

EKG artifact is common and can originate from the strong electrical field produced by cardiac activity, proximity to the field of the recording electrodes, or electrodes that are widely spaced (especially if the recording and reference electrodes cross the midline of the body). At times, EKG artifact occurring in the EEG may be mistaken fro abnormal brain electrical activity. In this recording, differentiation is based on several factors. Sharp activity only occurs in this one EEG channel, the sharp waves show no electrical field, and each corresponds with a QRS complex in the EKG. EKG artifact can occur in most recording channels, depending on filter settings.

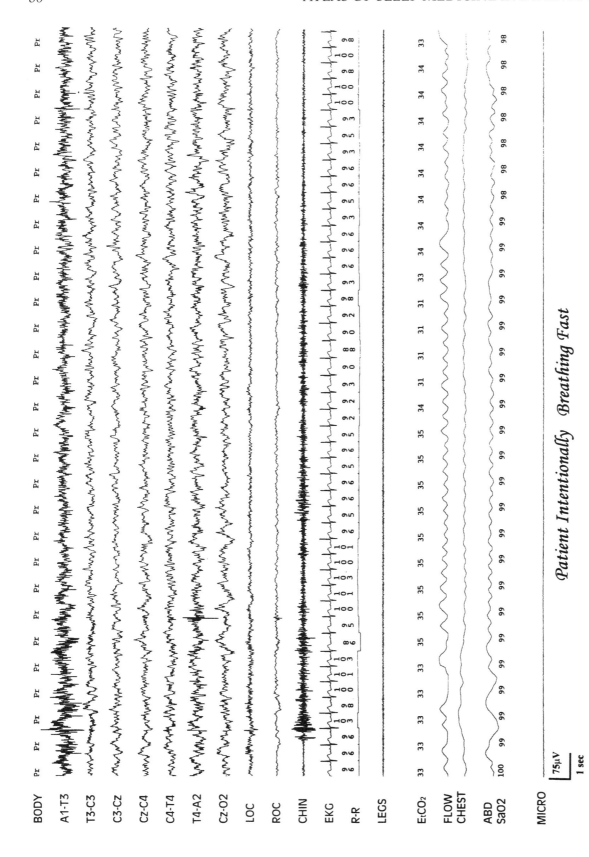

Patient Intentionally Breathing Fast

Intentional/Patient-Generated Artifact

Figure 29a. Intentional/Patient-Generated Artifact

This figure shows a polysomnographic segment recorded from a 6-year-old boy who was referred to the sleep medicine center for evaluation of sleep-disordered breathing. His tonsils were enlarged and he had a history of loud snoring and poor growth velocity. He was very cooperative during set-up and complied quite well with patient calibrations. Immediately after lights out, the following respiratory pattern was noted. EEG reveals a low voltage waking background frequency, muscle artifact in several EEG leads, and tonic chin muscle activity, but a respiratory rate of approximately 114 breaths per minute associated with relatively normal to slightly decreased E_tCO_2. Heart rate averages about 93 to 94 beats per minute. The technician noted in the record that the patient was intentionally breathing fast. Because tidal volume appeared to be quite low during this period of rapid respiration, hyperventilation with significant lowering of P_aCO_2 did not occur.

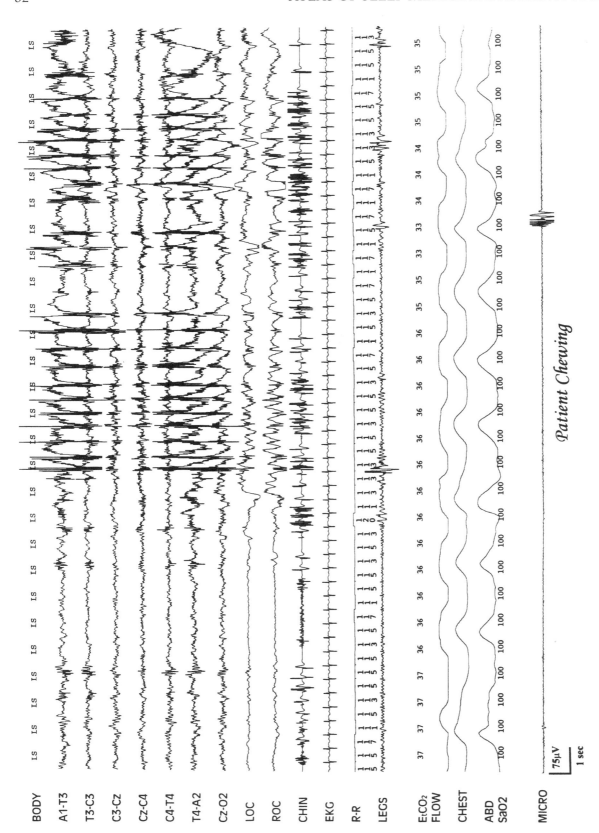

Patient Chewing

Intentional/Patient-Generated Artifact

Figure 29b. Intentional/Patient-Generated Artifact

This polysomnographic segment was recorded from the same patient after a prolonged arousal during the mid portion of the study and demonstrates rhythmic 1-Hz muscle artifact in the temporal regions of the EEG. Although this pattern of interference is characteristic of bruxism, it may be generated by chewing. The technician noted on the record that the patient woke and began to eat a piece of candy given to him by his mother.

Section IV

The Normal Polysomnogram in Infants and Children

The normal polysomnogram varies considerably as children mature. Polysomnographic changes that occur as a child ages have been termed *developmental polysomnography* and may provide useful information regarding neuro-developmental alterations over time. Anatomic and physiological reformations occur, sometimes very rapidly. At other times, neuro-developmental transformations are very slow.

There is wide variability between and within subjects studied in the pediatric sleep laboratory, and variation is the rule rather than the exception. Different strategies for polysomnographic evaluation and assessment are required for the pediatric patient.

The epochs and polysomnographic segments in this section illustrate classic features of the normal pediatric polysomnogram. Maturational perspectives are discussed. Stage 3 and stage 4 sleep have been consolidated into the single category of slow-wave sleep. Although categorization has been done by range of conceptional ages, examples from a single patient of a particular age group within each developmental period are provided. Principles discussed with each illustration are, nonetheless, consistent throughout each range.

Suggested Reading

1. Anders T, Emde R, Parmelee A (eds): *A Manual of Standardized Terminology, Techniques and Criteria for Scoring of States of Sleep and Wakefulness in Newborn Infants.* UCLA Brain Information Service, NINDS Neurological Information Network, 1971.
2. Bouterline-Young HJ, Smith CA: Respiration of full-term and of premature infants. Am J Dis Child 1953;80:753.
3. Daily WJR, Klaus M, Meyer HBP: Apnea in premature infants: Monitoring incidence, heart rate changes, and effect of environmental temperature. Pediatrics 1969;43:510–518.
4. Dransfield DA, Spiter AR, Fox WW: Episodic airway obstruction in premature infants. Am J Dis Child 1983;137:441–443.
5. Eliaschar I, Lavie P, Halperen E, et al: Sleep apneic episodes as indications for adenotonsillectomy. Arch Otolaryngol 1980;106:492–496.
6. Feinberg I: Eye movement activity during sleep and intellectual function in mental retardation. Science 1968;159:1256.
7. Ferber R: *Solve Your Child's Sleep Problems.* New York: Simon & Schuster, 1985.
8. Hertz G, Cataletto M, Feinsilver SH, et al: Sleep and breathing patterns in patients with Prader Willi syndrome (PWS): Effects of age and gender. Sleep 1993;16:366–371.
9. Kahn A, Dan B, Groswasser J, et al: Normal sleep architecture in infants and children. J Clin Neurophysiol 1996;13(3):184–197.
10. Kahn A, Rebuffat E, Sottiaux M, et al: Arousals induced by proximal esophageal reflux in infants. Sleep 1991;14:39–42.
11. Karni A, Tanne D, Rubenstein BS, et al: Dependence on REM sleep of overnight improvement of a perceptual skill. Science 1994;265:679–682.
12. Milner AD, Boon AW, Saunders RA, et al: Upper airway obstruction and apnea in preterm babies. Arch Dis Child 1980;55:22–25.

13. National Institutes of Health Consensus Development Conference: *Infantile Apnea and Home Monitoring.* Bethesda, MD: US Department of Health and Human Services, Oct 1, 1987, NIH Pub. No. 87-2905.
14. Paul K, Dittrichova J: Sleep patterns following learning in infants. In Levin P, Koella U (eds): *Sleep: 1974.* Basel: S Karger, 1975, p. 388.
15. Kellaway P, Petersen I (eds): *Clinical Electroencephalography of Children.* New York: Grune & Stratton, 1968.
16. Parmelee AH Jr, Schulte FJ, Akiyama Y, et al: Maturation of EEG activity during sleep in premature infants. Electroenceph Clin Neurophysiol 1968;24:319–329.
17. Petre-Quaden O: Ontogenesis of paradoxical sleep in the human newborn. J Neurol Sci 1967;4:153.
18. Rechtschaffen A, Kales A (eds): *A Manual of Standardized Terminology, Techniques and Scoring System for Sleep Stages of Human Subjects.* Los Angeles: BIS/BRI, UCLA, 1968.
19. Rigatto H: Apnea. Pediatr Clin North Am 1982;29:1105–1116.
20. Ross RJ, Ball WA, Dinges DF, et al: Motor dysfunction during sleep in post-traumatic stress disorder. Sleep 1994;17:723–732.
21. Rowe P (ed): *The Harriet Lane Handbook.* Chicago: Year Book, 1987, p. 64.
22. Sheldon SH: *Evaluating Sleep in Infants and Children.* New York: Lippincott-Raven, 1996.
23. Sheldon SH, Ahart S, Levy HB: Sleep patterns in abused and neglected children. Sleep Res 1991;20:333.
24. Sheldon SH, Jacobsen J: REM sleep motor disorder in children. J Child Neurol 1998;3:257–260.
25. Sheldon SH, Irbe D, Applebaum J, et al: Sleep pressure in children with attentional deficits. Sleep Res 1991;20A:448.
26. Sheldon SH, Jacobsen J: REM-sleep motor disorder in children. J Child Neurol 1998;13:257–260.
27. Sheldon SH, Onal E, Lilie J, et al: Sleep-related post-inspiratory upper-airway obstruction in children. Sleep Res 1993;22:270.
28. Sheldon SH, Spire JP, Levy HB: *Pediatric Sleep Medicine.* Philadelphia: WB Saunders, 1992.
29. Sheldon SH, Spire JP, Levy HB: REM sleep eye movements in reading disabled children. Sleep Res 1990;19:128.
30. Silverman A, Roy CC: *Pediatric Clinical Gastroenterology.* St Louis: CV Mosby Company, 1983, pp. 149–151.
31. Spehlmann R: *EEG Primer.* Amsterdam, The Netherlands: Elsevier, 1981.
32. Thach BT, Stark AR: Spontaneous neck flexion and airway obstruction during apneic spells in preterm infants. J Pediatr 1979;94:275–281.
33. Tirosh E, Sadeh A, Munvez R, et al: Effects of methylphenidate on sleep in children with attention-deficit hyperactivity disorder: An activity monitor study. Am J Dis Child 1993;147:1313–1315.
34. Wilson MA, McNaughton BL: Reactivation of hippocampal ensemble memories during sleep. Science 1994;265:676–679.
35. Winter HS: Gastroesophageal reflux. In Rudolph AM, Hoffman JIE (eds): *Pediatrics.* 18th ed. Norwalk, Connecticut: Appleton Lange, 1987, pp. 906–908.

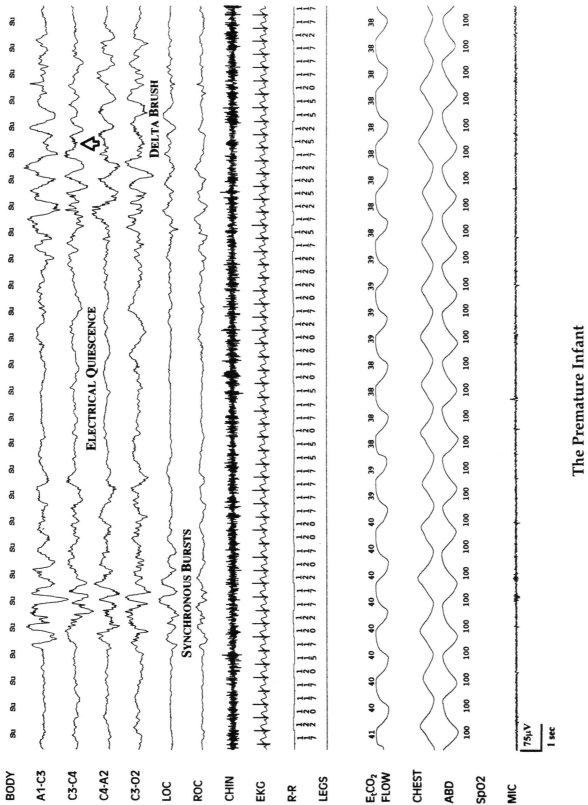

The Premature Infant

Figure 30a. The Premature Infant

Prior to 28 weeks' gestation, sleep and wake activity cannot be clearly identified electrographically. EEG consists of periods of no activity which may last up to 3 minutes. This inactivity is separated by intermittent bursts of activity lasting about 20 seconds. Bursts are usually bilaterally synchronous. After 28 weeks' conceptional age, an EEG pattern of tracé discontinué appears. This pattern is characterized by discontinuous activity of rhythmic waves, lasting 1 to 2 seconds at a frequency of approximately 4 to 6 Hz. Fast waves of about 10 to 20 Hz appear superimposed on slow waves (0.5 to 1 Hz) and continue until shortly before conceptional term. This fast activity is termed delta brushes.

Between 32 and 36 weeks' conceptional age, the discontinuous pattern of 1- to 2-Hz slow waves continues and is mostly concentrated over the posterior regions of the head. A new pattern of continuous slow wave activity begins to appear during periods of wakefulness and active sleep. More than 85% of the total sleep time during this developmental stage comprises this active sleep.

This figure shows a recording from a 36-week-old premature male who had mild respiratory distress syndrome, required ventilation for about 48 hours, and was subsequently extubated without complications. Between 36 weeks' conceptional age and term, there is continuous development and modification of EEG and polysomnographic patterns. The discontinuous pattern now has shorter pauses and low amplitude waves may appear between the bursts of slow waves. This EEG pattern is termed tracé alternant and is characteristic of quiet sleep. Delta brushes can still be seen in this recording. During quiet sleep chin muscle tone may be slightly decreased, but it remains tonic. Sucking movements may be noted. Little phasic activity is present and eye movements are absent. Respiratory pattern is very regular and monotonous.

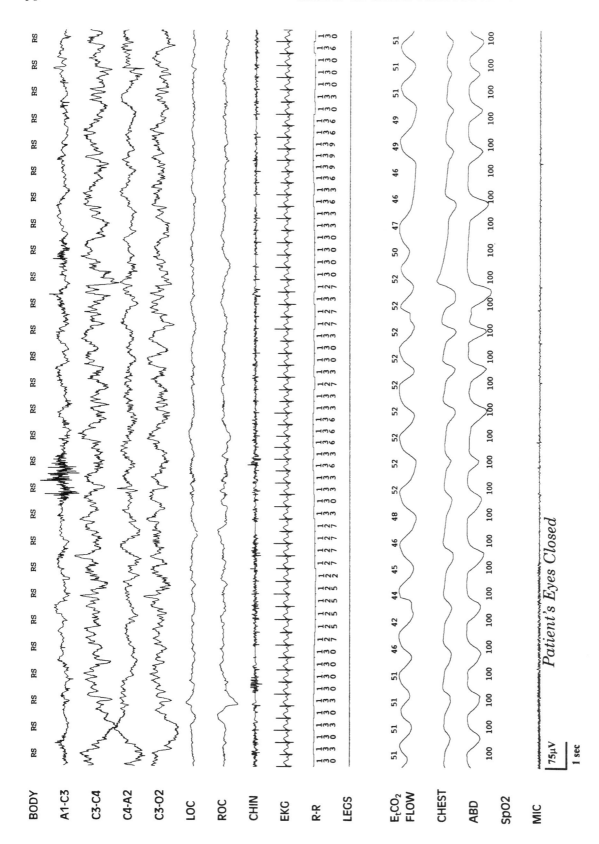

The Premature Infant

Figure 30b. The Premature Infant

This figure shows a recording from the patient in Figure 30a, and demonstrates continuous irregular slow waves in the theta and delta frequency and diffuse irregular continuous slow waves of relatively low amplitude (<50 μV), a pattern now characteristically seen during wakefulness and active sleep. Active sleep is associated with continuous moderately low voltage EEG activity associated with decreased chin muscle tone, intense phasic and motor activity, and conjugate eye movements. Respiratory pattern is very irregular, brief apneas and hypopneas are common, and periodic breathing is typical. The amount of total sleep time occupied by periodic breathing decreases considerably as conceptional term approaches. Gross body movements, facial and limb twitches, and vocalizations are normal during active sleep. Since similar EEG and motor patterns may occur during both wakefulness and active sleep, polysomnographic state determination is often difficult. Technician notation of behavioral characteristics is required to assist the polysomnographer in determination of state. *Sustained eye closure is most reliable in determining sleep in premature and young infants. It is therefore important for the technician to frequently document on the recording whether the infant's eyes are open or closed.*

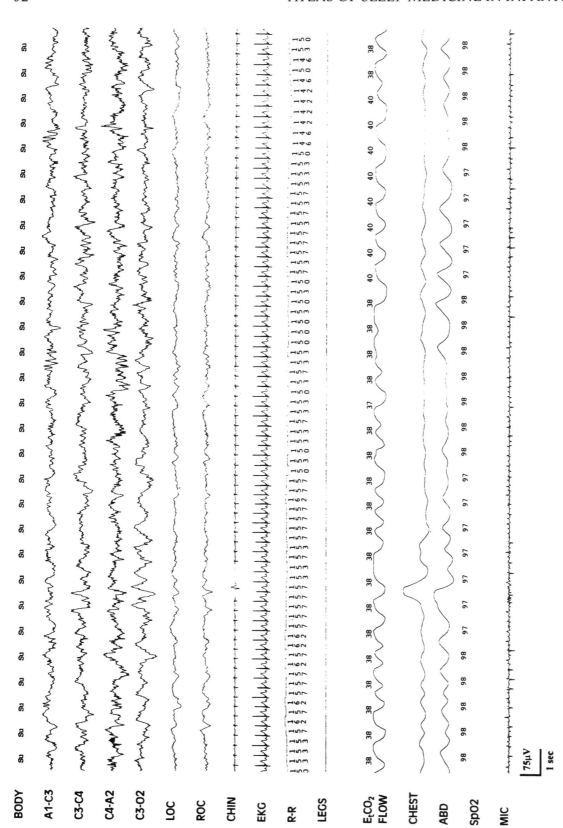

The Premature Infant

Figure 30c. The Premature Infant

The polysomnographic segment in this figure was recorded from the same 36-week conceptional-age infant. Characteristics of both active and quiet sleep are present in this polysomnographic segment. The term *indeterminate sleep* has been used to described a state where neither active nor quiet sleep could be adequately identified. Indeterminate sleep appears to demonstrate state dissociation. Some data exist that suggest that increased percent of state dissociation occurring after conceptional term may be an indicator of neuro-developmental outcome.

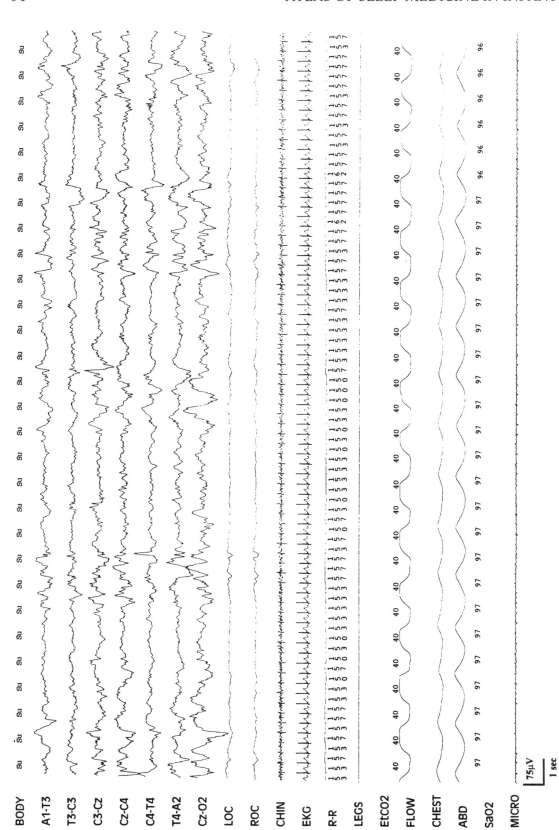

The Infant at Conceptional Term

Figure 31a. The Infant at Conceptional Term

This figure shows a recording from a 3-day-old term male infant with left choanal atresia and right choanal stenosis, who was referred for evaluation of stridulous breathing during sleep. In this segment, normal quiet sleep is demonstrated. At 40 weeks' conceptional age, the predominant EEG pattern seen during quiet sleep is *tracé alternant*. Note the discontinuous pattern of high amplitude slow waves lasting several seconds, alternating with low amplitude activity also lasting several seconds. Bursts of activity are synchronous. Delta brushes are no longer present, and occasional slow waves are seen between bursts. This pattern gradually disappears between 40 and 44 weeks' conceptional age. EOG reveals no significant eye movements. Heart rate is very regular with some beat-to-beat variability. Respiratory pattern is also quite regular. Paradoxical pattern of chest and abdominal movements during breathing is normal during infancy due to increased chest wall compliance. Chest and abdominal efforts that are out of phase during infancy do not necessarily imply airway obstruction or respiratory distress.

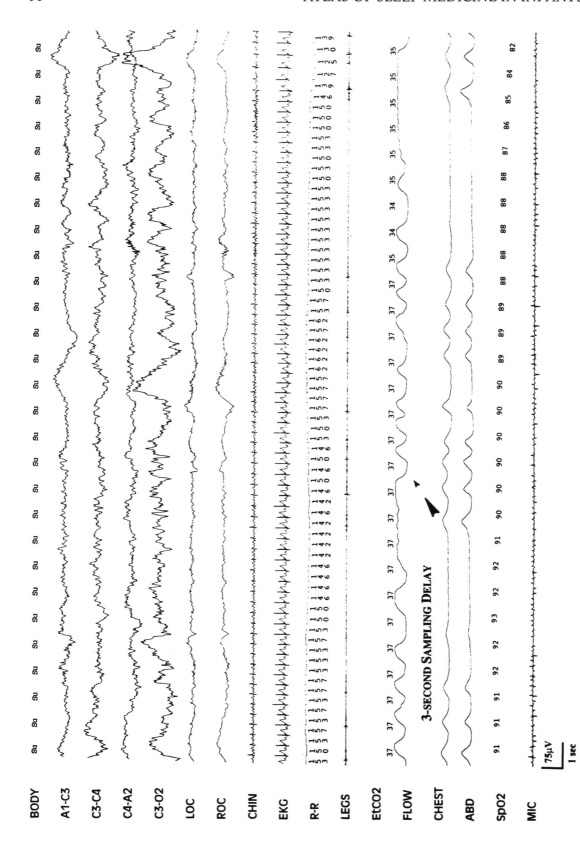

The Infant at Conceptional Term

Figure 31b. The Infant at Conceptional Term

This polysomnographic segment was recorded during active sleep from a 1-day-old term newborn who was being evaluated for unexplained periods of oxygen desaturation during sleep. Periodic breathing was noted by her nurses, but there were no color changes. Heart rate remained stable and no prolonged apneas were noted.

Active sleep may appear quite similar polysomnographically to wakefulness in young infants. There is considerable motor activity, intermixed with periods of quiescence. Newborn infants typically enter sleep through active sleep, and the exact transition into sleep is based on the appearance of a characteristic polysomnographic pattern *and the technician's notation that the baby has sustained eye closure.* There is diffuse 1- to 2-Hz continuous activity, which is rhythmic and synchronous. Although muscle tone is decreased during active sleep, there are superimposed major body movements, muscle phasic activity, twitches, facial grimaces, smiles, and vocalizations. EOG reveals rapid saccades of eye movements. Respiration is irregular and there may be periodic breathing during active sleep. Note periodic breathing and moderate oxygen desaturation to a low of 81%. Hypopneas and brief apneas are common. The younger the conceptional age, the greater the percent of periodic breathing and indeterminate sleep.

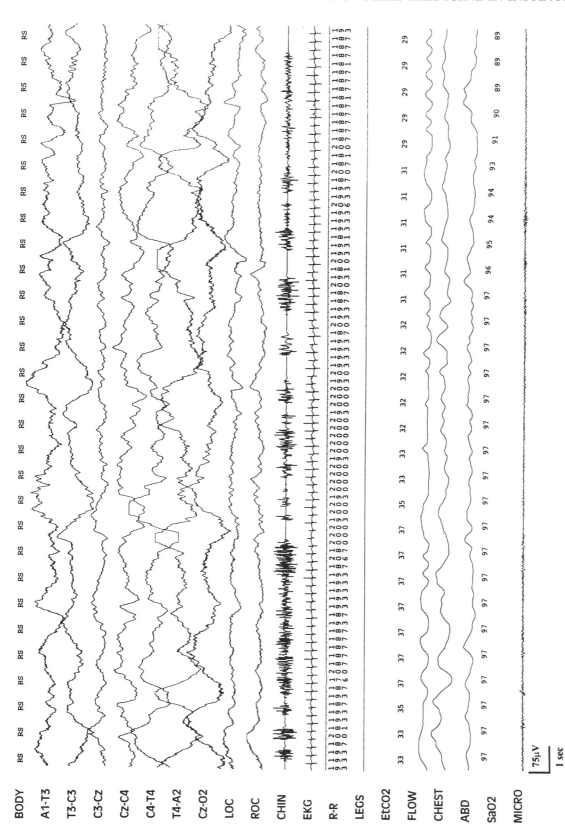

Normal Sleep in a 2-Month-Old Infant

Figure 32a. Normal Sleep in a 2-Month-Old Infant

This figure represents a polysomnographic segment recorded during wakefulness from a 2-month-old infant who was referred for evaluation of frequent nocturnal awakenings and noisy breathing during sleep. EEG consists of continuous activity, as well as considerable movement and sweat artifact. Chin EMG reveals intermittent increases and decreases in tone produced as the infant nurses. Heart rate is elevated and respiratory channels demonstrate irregularities of breathing associated with nursing. Decrease seen in airflow near the center of the epoch is associated with swallowing. Movement associated with this pause in respiration resulted in a decrease in oxygen saturation.

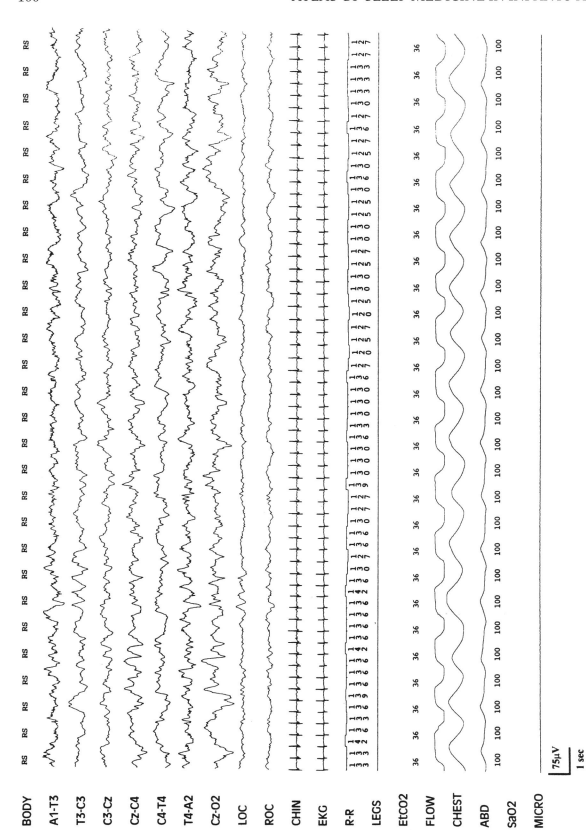

Normal Sleep in a 2-Month-Old Infant

Figure 32b. Normal Sleep in a 2-Month-Old Infant

The segment shown here was recorded from the same patient during quiet sleep. EEG reveals slow waves and superimposed theta activity. Heart rate has decreased from that seen during wakefulness, and respiratory pattern is very regular.

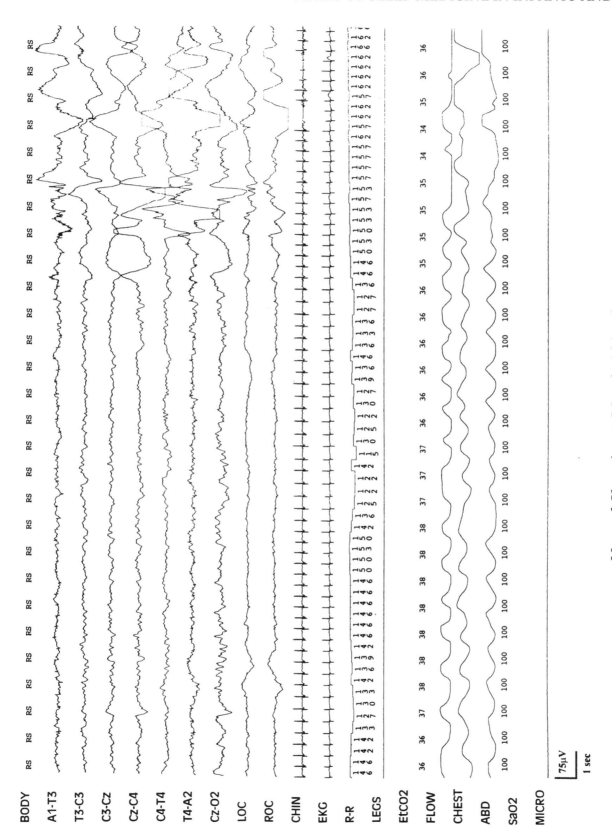

Normal Sleep in a 2-Month-Old Infant

Figure 32c. Normal Sleep in a 2-Month-Old Infant

This figure shows a recording from the same infant during active sleep. Lower amplitude EEG is present. The heart rate is higher than during quiet sleep and there is more heart rate variability. Considerable irregularity in breathing is present, indicating normal respiratory instability during active sleep. A gross body movement is present near the end of the epoch. Gross movements, twitches, grimaces, arm and leg movements, sucking, and vocalizations are common and normal during active sleep in infants during this developmental period.

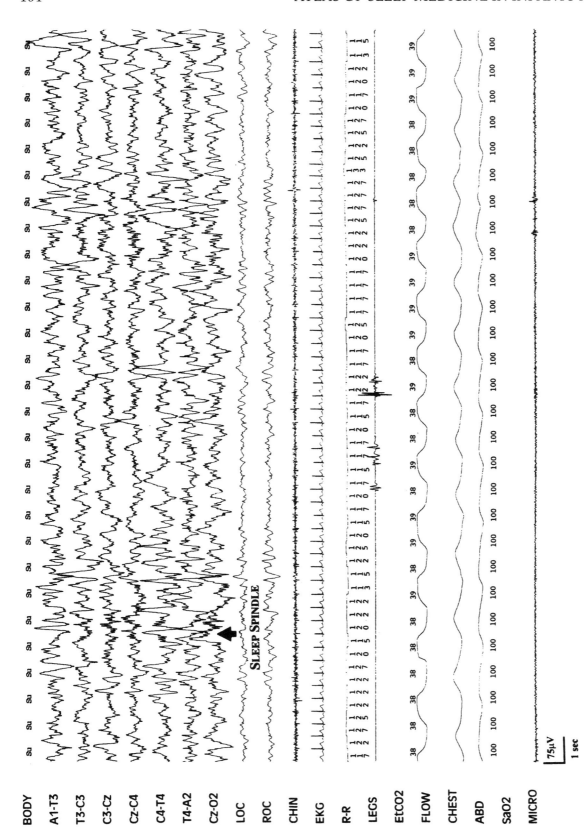

Normal Sleep in a 4-Month-Old Infant

to become evident in the EEG pattern when compared to earlier developmental periods. Faster frequency and lower voltage activity are present, along with long sleep spindles. NREM sleep in infants younger than 1 year of age is often "scored" as quiet sleep. If state differentiation is clear, however, sleep stages may be scored as in older children.

Figure 33a. Normal Sleep in a 4-Month-Old Infant

This is a recording that was taken during quiet sleep from a 4-month-old infant who was referred for evaluation of a cyanotic episode during sleep that was witnessed by his parents. The youngster was born at term and was otherwise healthy. He had received immunizations 1 week prior to the cyanotic episode. Differences start

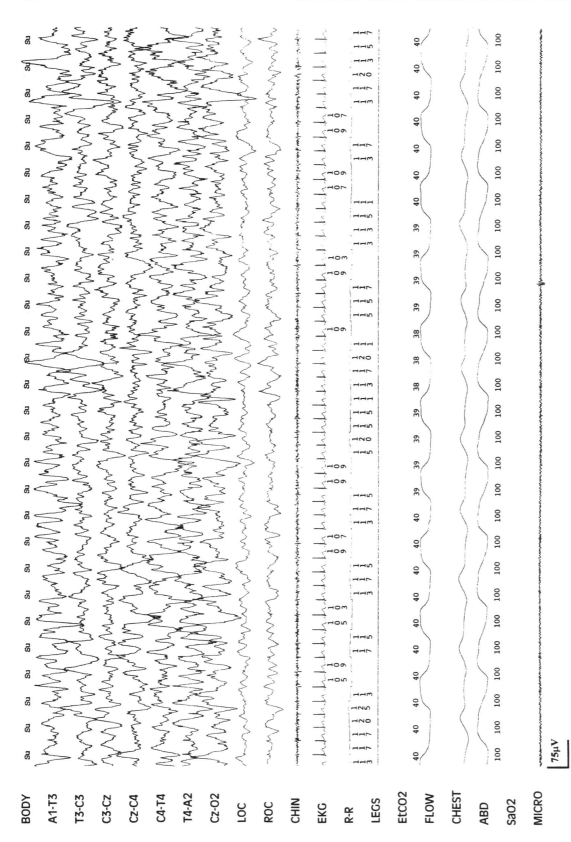

Normal Sleep in a 4-Month-Old Infant

Figure 33b. Normal Sleep in a 4-Month-Old Infant

This is a recording from the infant shown in Figure 33a during quiet sleep. Although Figures 33a and 33b might appear similar, this figure reveals a slower background activity of greater amplitude. There are fewer noticeable sleep spindles and there is increased EEG artifact in the EOG. Relatively steady heart rate and regular respiratory patterns with normal E_tCO_2 and oxygen saturation can be seen in both polysomnographic segments.

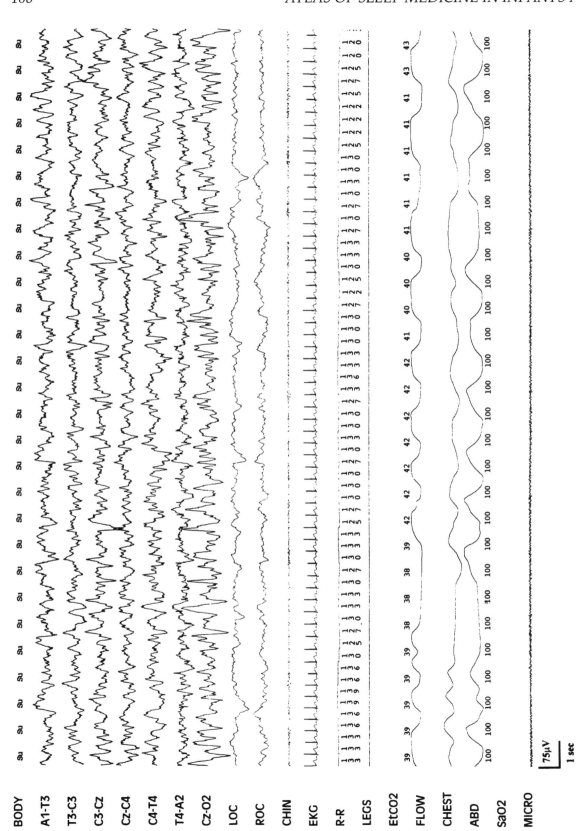

Normal Sleep in a 4-Month-Old Infant

.

Figure 33c. Normal Sleep in a 4-Month-Old Infant

This figure shows a recording from the same patient during REM/active sleep. EEG reveals moderate voltage continuous activity with a mixture of theta and delta frequencies. Conjugate rapid eye movements can be seen in the EOG, and chin tone is significantly decreased below the levels seen in the previous two segments. Heart rate is regular, but faster than during NREM sleep. Respiratory pattern shows irregular effort, and a brief (normal) central apnea is present near the beginning of the epoch.

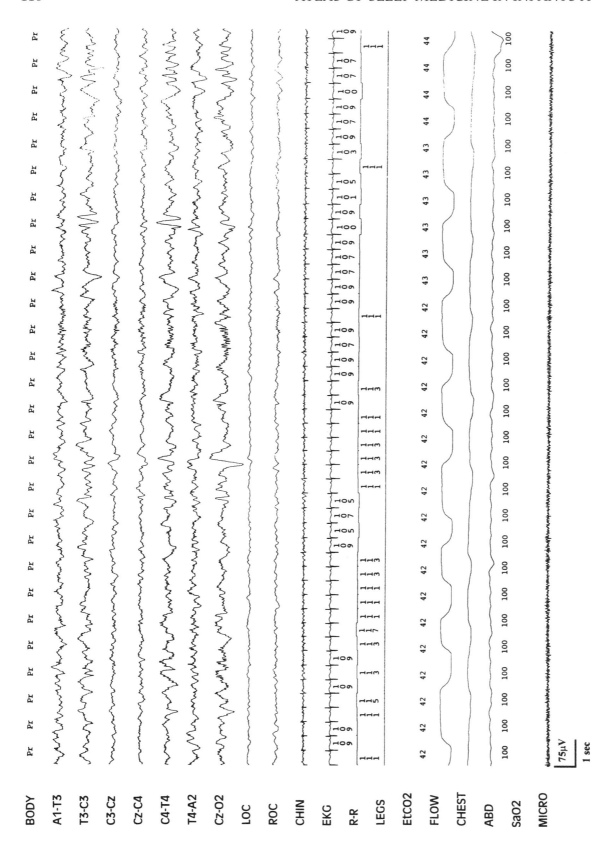

Normal Sleep in a 7-Month-Old Infant

Figure 34a. Normal Sleep in a 7-Month-Old Infant

The polysomnographic segment shown in here was recorded during NREM sleep from a 7-month-old, apparently normal, term infant whose sibling had died of sudden infant death syndrome at 3 months of age. There is now clear differentiation between stage 2 sleep and SWS. A relatively low voltage background EEG activity is seen and synchronous sleep spindles are easily visible. Eye movements are absent and Chin EMG is tonic. Respiration is very regular. E_tCO_2 and oxygen saturation are normal. Heart rate reveals normal beat-to-beat variability.

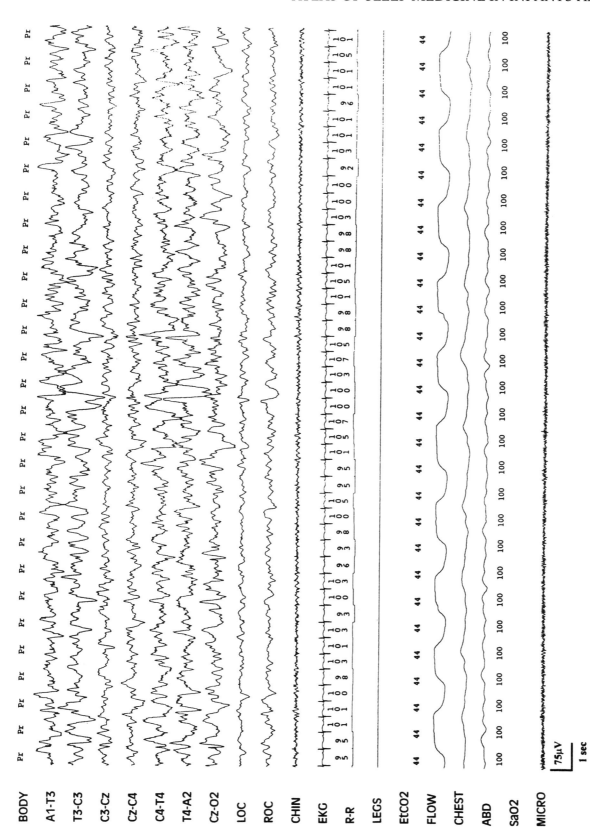

Normal Sleep in a 7-Month-Old Infant

Figure 34b. Normal Sleep in a 7-Month-Old Infant

This figure shows a recording that was taken during SWS. There is a low frequency, high amplitude EEG. EEG artifact is seen in the EOG channels due to high EEG voltage. Heart rate is somewhat slower than seen in stage 2.

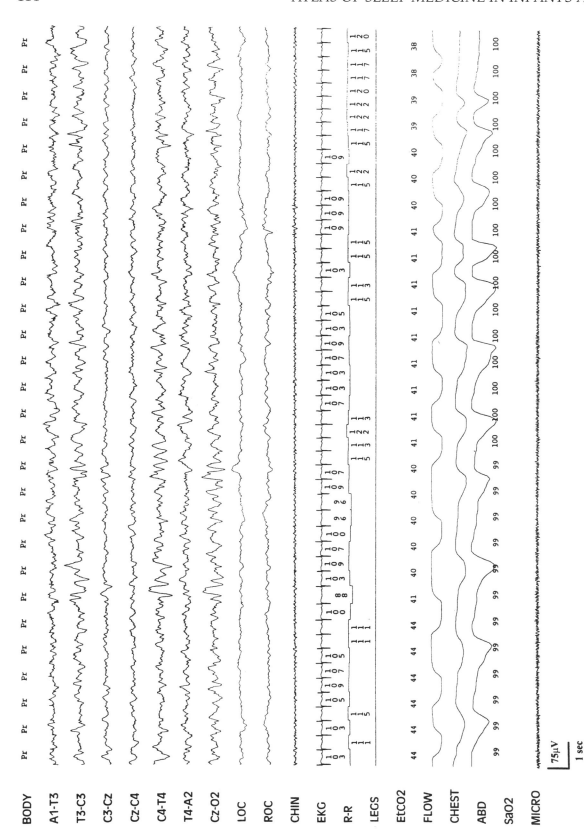

Normal Sleep in a 7-Month-Old Infant

Figure 34c. Normal Sleep in a 7-Month-Old Infant

This polysomnographic segment was recorded during REM sleep. EEG reveals relatively high voltage theta and delta activity. Conjugate eye movements are present in the EOG. Respiratory pattern and heart rate are more variable than during NREM sleep. Oxygen saturation and E_tCO_2 continue to be normal.

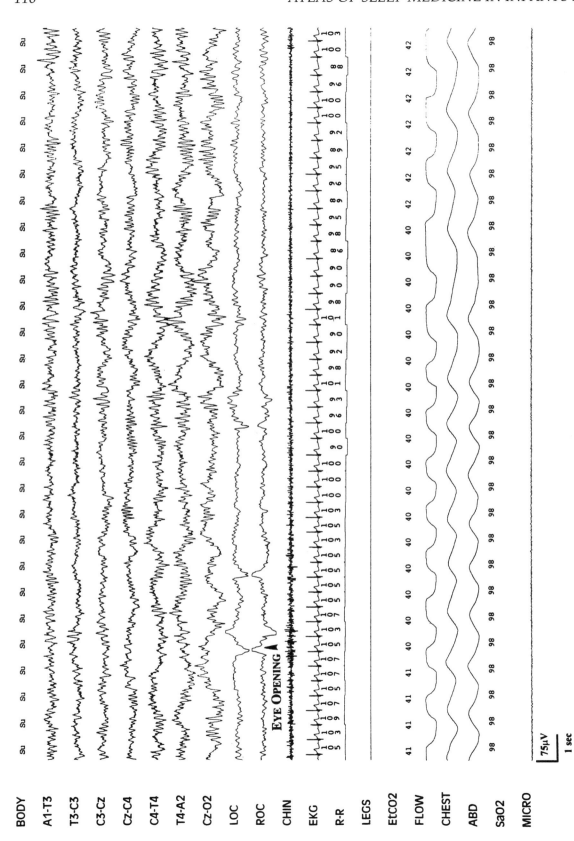

Normal Wake in a 17-Month-Old-Toddler

Figure 35a. Normal Wake in a 17-Month-Old-Toddler

The segment shown in here was recorded during wakefulness from a 17-month-old toddler who was referred as part of an evaluation for failure-to-thrive. His weight was only 6 kg and there was a history of loud snoring and very restless sleep. He woke frequently during the night. In this segment, there is a moderate amplitude 5- to 6-Hz EEG background. During the brief period of eye opening, there is a decrease in amplitude and an increase in frequency of the EEG. Conjugate eye movements are noted and relatively high chin tone helps identify this epoch as wake.

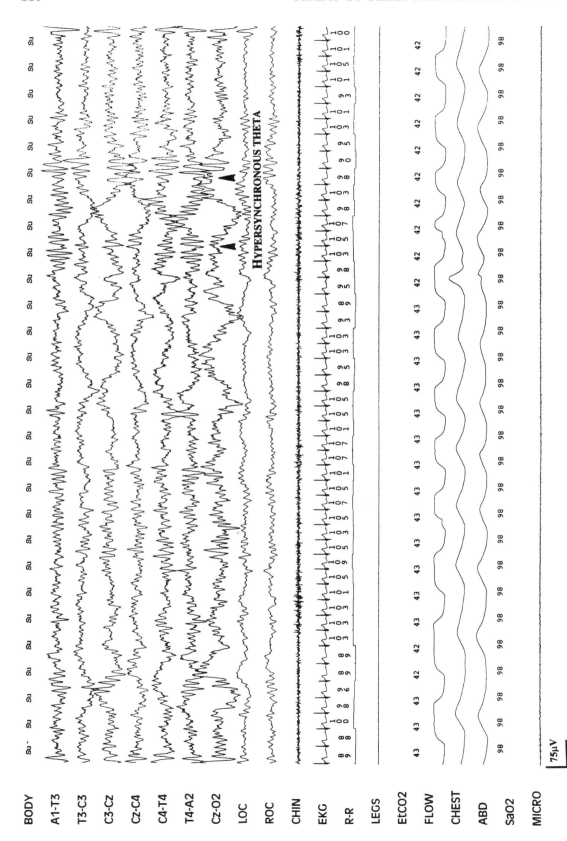

Normal Sleep in a 17-Month-Old-Toddler

Figure 35b. Normal Sleep in a 17-Month-Old-Toddler

The recording shown in this figure represents transition from wake to sleep. EEG reveals bursts of hypersynchronous 4- to 5-Hz, high amplitude waveforms. These bursts of hypersynchronous activity early during the sleep period may appear quite sharp, but they are a normal finding over the vertex during this developmental period. EOG shows slow rolling eye movements. Chin muscle is tonic. EKG and respiratory pattern are relatively stable.

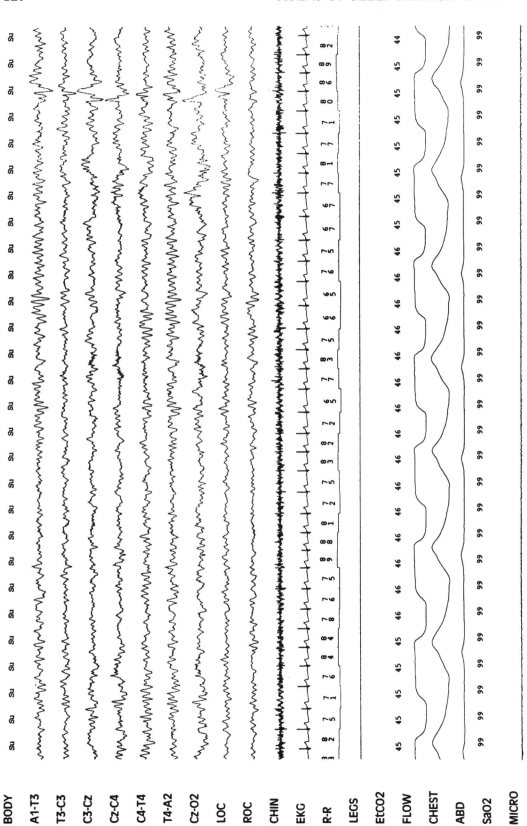

Normal Sleep in a 17-Month-Old-Toddler

Figure 35c. Normal Sleep in a 17-Month-Old-Toddler

The polysomnographic segment shown in this figure represents normal stage 2 sleep. A relatively moderate voltage, mixed frequency EEG background is noted. Sleep spindles are present and symmetrical. Chin EMG continues to remain tonic, heart rate has slowed when compared to sleep onset, and normal respiratory sinus variation is present. Respiratory pattern is regular. Oxygen saturation and E_tCO_2 are normal.

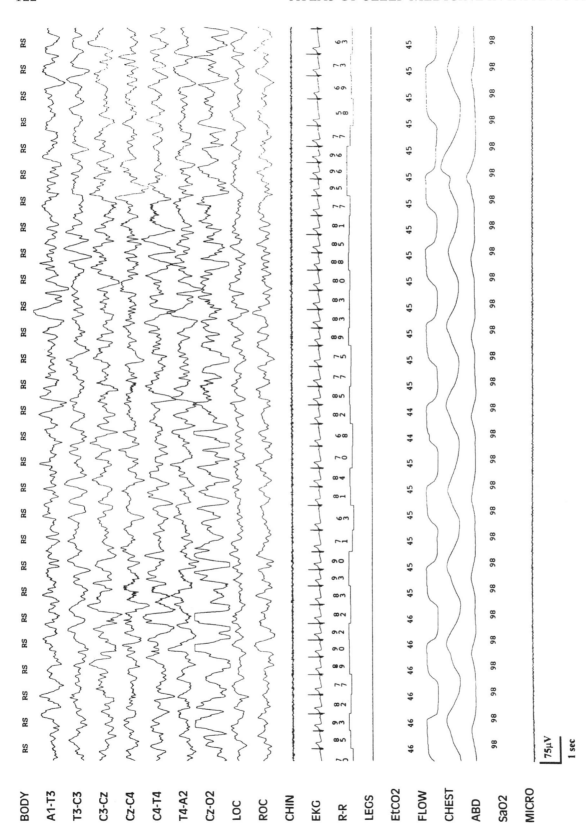

Normal Sleep in a 17-Month-Old-Toddler

Figure 35d. Normal Sleep in a 17-Month-Old-Toddler

The polysomnographic recording shown here depicts SWS. EEG is dominated by high voltage waves of 1 to 2 Hz. Sleep spindles are present and superimposed on the slow wave activity. EOG reveals considerable EEG artifact due to the high amplitude of the frontal EEG activity. Heart rate shows a sinus arrhythmia, and respiratory patterns are regular with normal oxygen saturation and E_tCO_2.

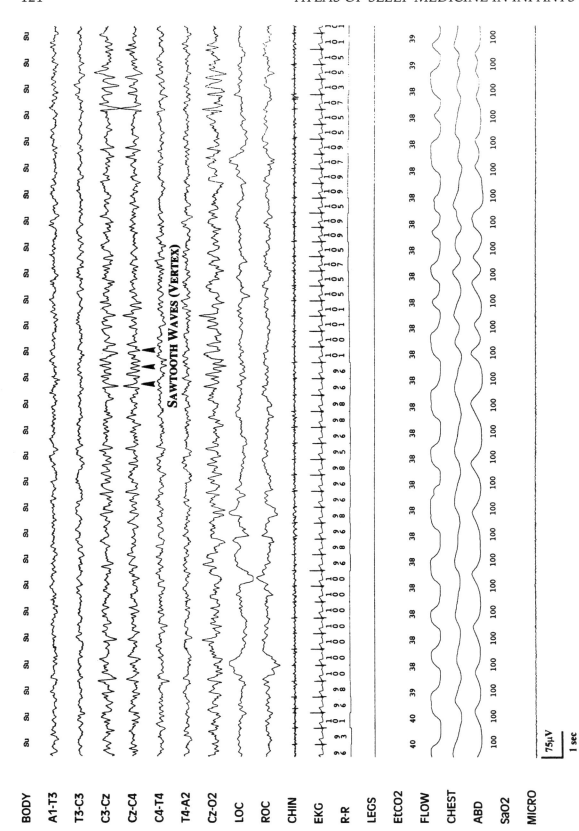

Normal Sleep in a 17-Month-Old-Toddler

Figure 35e. Normal Sleep in a 17-Month-Old-Toddler

This figure demonstrates REM sleep. EEG consists of moderate amplitude, notched, theta activity (sawtooth waves), particularly over the vertex. Clear conjugate eye movements are present in the EOG. Chin tone is decreased compared to all prior polysomnogram segments. Heart rate is similar to that of wakefulness. There is marked irregularity in respiratory effort, but oxygen saturation and E_tCO_2 remain normal. There is paradoxical movement of the chest and abdomen, as is normally seen in young children during REM sleep. This is due to increased compliance of the rib cage from normal decrease in tone of accessory muscles of respiration.

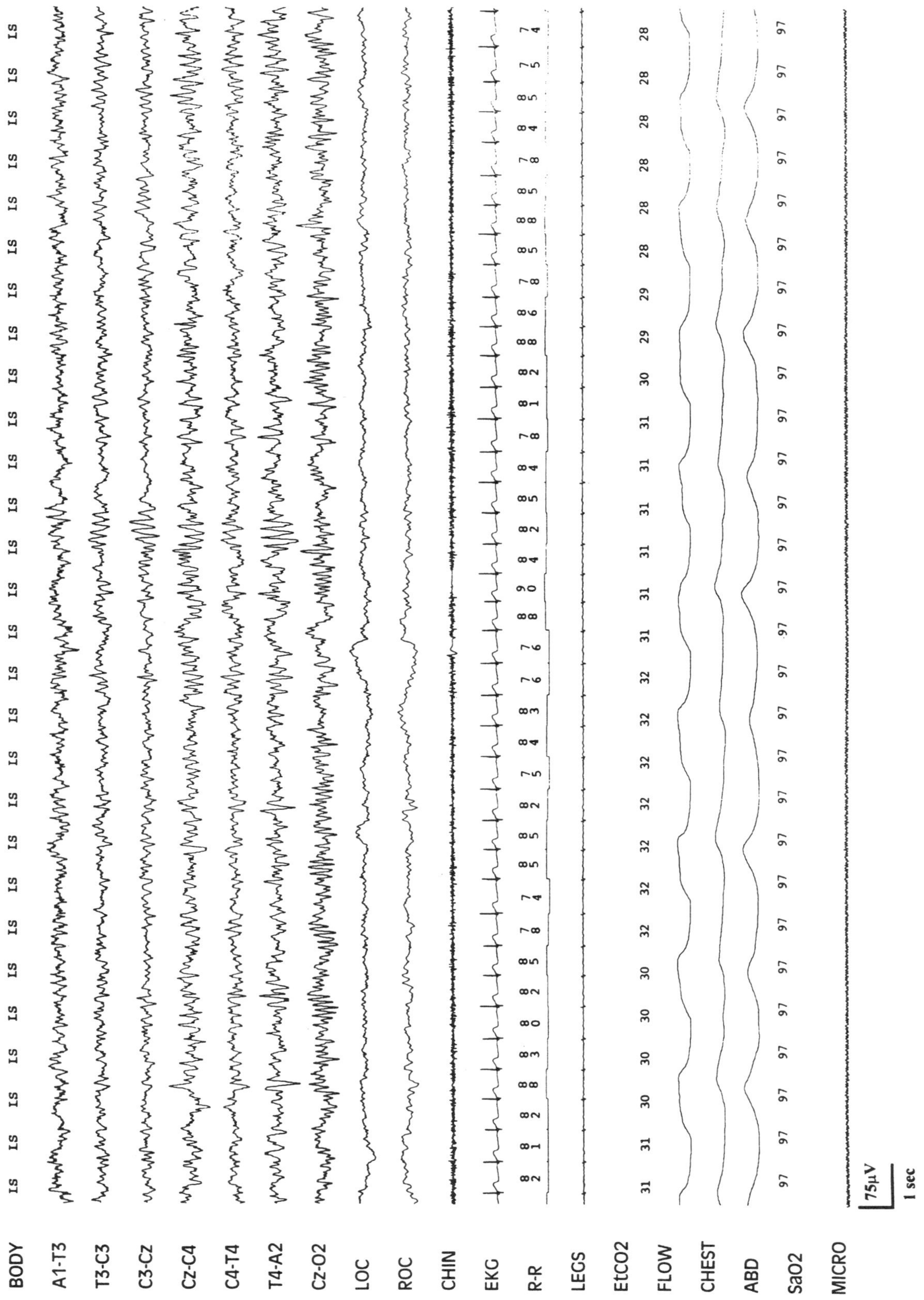

BODY

A1-T3

T3-C3

C3-Cz

Cz-C4

C4-T4

T4-A2

Cz-O2

LOC

ROC

CHIN

EKG

R-R

LEGS

EtCO2

FLOW

CHEST

ABD

SaO2

MICRO

75μV

1 sec

Normal Wake in a 3-Year-Old Child

Figure 36a. Normal Wake in a 3-Year-Old Child

This polysomnographic recording was obtained during transition from wake to sleep in a 3-year-old child who had been referred for evaluation of possible sleep-disordered breathing. Waking EEG background frequency is 6 to 7 Hz. Frequency begins to slow to approximately 4 to 6 Hz and amplitude increases to about 100 µV. A transition from conjugate eye movements to slow, rolling move-

ments occurs. Chin muscle is tonic, although there is brief decreased tone during the transition to sleep. Heart rate is stable, there are no limb movements, and regular chest and abdominal efforts with good airflow can be seen. In this segment, E_tCO_2 is slightly low, which may be due to slight displacement of the sampling cannula after a body movement prior to sleep onset. Oxygen saturation is normal and there is no snoring recorded sonographically.

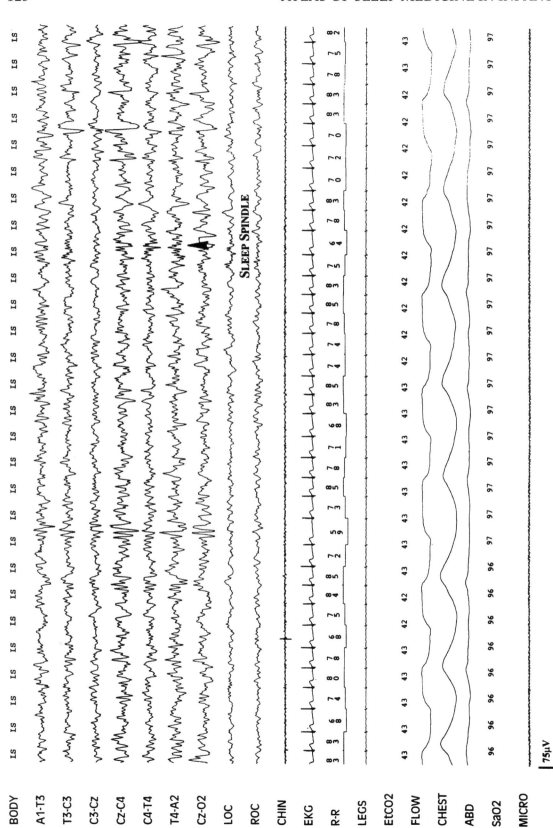

Normal Sleep in a 3-Year-Old Child

Figure 36b. Normal Sleep in a 3-Year-Old Child

This figure represents stage 2 sleep. There is mixed 2- to 6-Hz background EEG activity with sleep spindles at a frequency of approximately 14 Hz. No eye movements are recorded on EOG. EKG shows a normal sinus arrhythmia with a slower rate than that seen during wake. All respiratory channels are normal, with restoration of a good flow signal in the nasal/oral channel. E_tCO_2 is within a normal range.

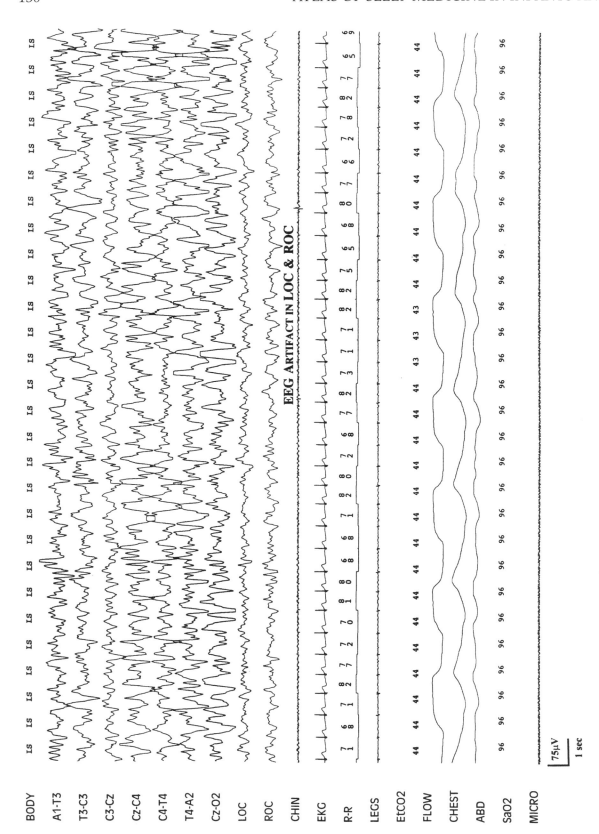

Normal Sleep in a 3-Year-Old Child

Figure 36c. Normal Sleep in a 3-Year-Old Child

This polysomnographic segment was recorded during SWS. EEG demonstrates high amplitude 0.5- to 2-Hz activity occupying more than 50% of this 30-second epoch. Movement in the EOG reflects high amplitude frontal EEG activity. Chin tone is relatively low. Cardiac rhythm shows normal sinus variation with breathing. Rate is slightly slower than that seen during stage 2 or wake. All respiratory channels demonstrate normal breathing.

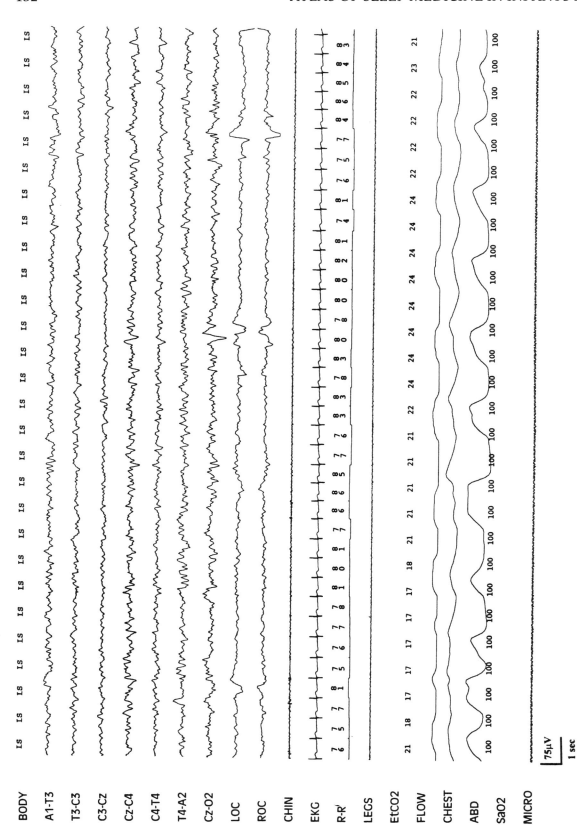

Normal Sleep in a 3-Year-Old Child

Figure 36d. Normal Sleep in a 3-Year-Old Child

This figure represents REM sleep. Moderate amplitude theta EEG activity, rapid conjugate eye movements, increased heart rate over NREM sleep states, and low chin muscle tone are present. Respiratory channels reveal a characteristic irregular breathing pattern. Some paradoxical movements are noted in the chest and abdomen. Oxygen saturation is normal. E_tCO_2 is low in the presence of normal oxygen saturation and respiratory rate, suggesting that the patient has displaced the cannula to a less than optimal position.

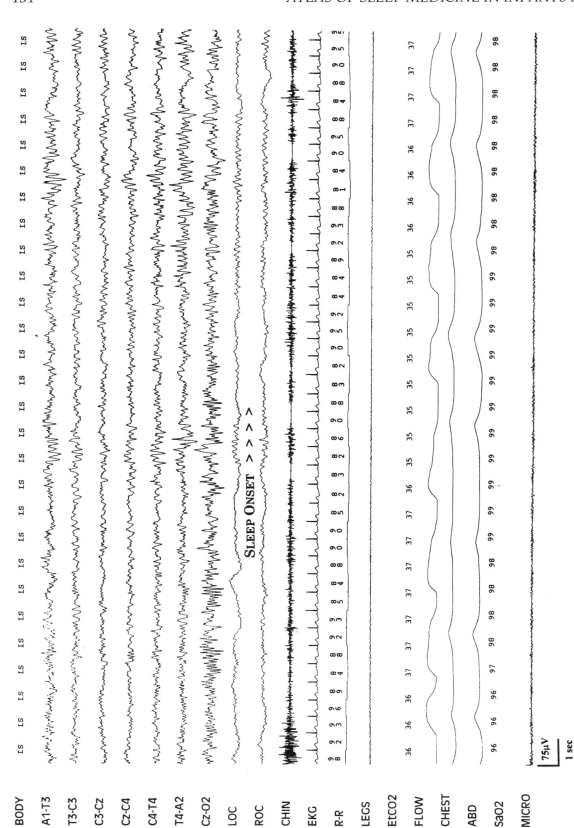

Normal Sleep in a 7-Year-Old Male

Figure 37a. Normal Sleep in a 7-Year-Old Male

This figure demonstrates transition from wake to sleep in a 7-year-old male who was admitted to the hospital for exacerbation of reactive airways disease. He was treated with nebulized albuterol and steroids with good resolution of symptoms. The night prior to discharge, nurses noted loud snoring without oxygen desaturations. A well-formed alpha rhythm of approximately 9 Hz is demonstrated and concentrated over the occipital region (Cz-O2). EEG rhythm slows to a predominantly theta rhythm of about 5 Hz.

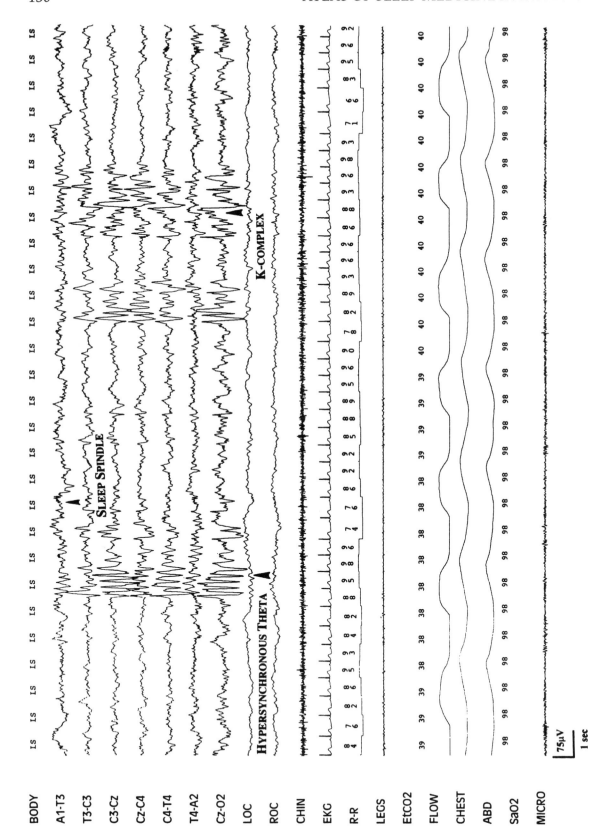

Normal Sleep in a 7-Year-Old Male

Figure 37b. Normal Sleep in a 7-Year-Old Male

This polysomnographic recording shows further transition into NREM sleep, and the appearance of stage 2 sleep. Note the bursts of hypersynchronous theta activity. K complexes and sleep spindles appear.

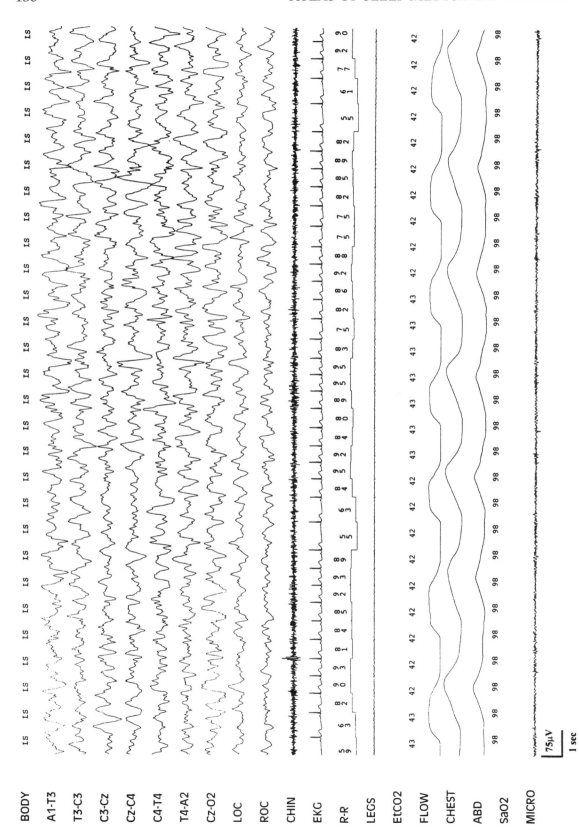

Normal Sleep in a 7-Year-Old Male

Figure 37c. Normal Sleep in a 7-Year-Old Male

The polysomnographic segment in this figure was recorded during SWS. EEG consists of very high voltage (>250 μV), 0.5- to 1-Hz activity. Normal respiratory variability in the heart rate can be seen.

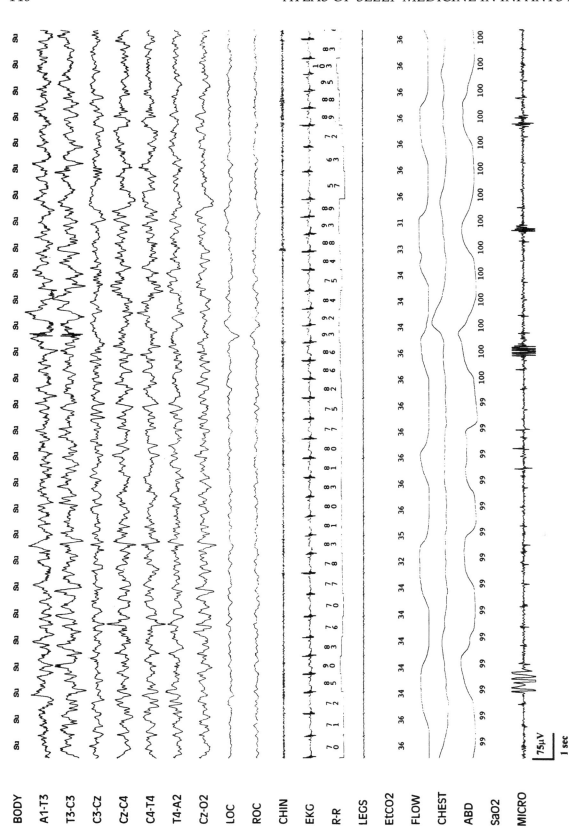

Normal Sleep in a 7-Year-Old Male

Figure 37d. Normal Sleep in a 7-Year-Old Male

This figure was recorded from the same patient, in REM sleep. EEG consists of relatively low voltage, mixed frequency waveforms and sawtooth waves. Rapid conjugate eye movements are present and chin tone is low. Respiration is irregular with normal oxygen saturation and E_tCO_2. Snoring is present in the sonogram.

Section V

The Abnormal Polysomnogram in Infants and Children

The following polysomnographic segments have been collected from the archives of the Sleep Medicine Center at The Children's Memorial Hospital, Chicago. Epochs are, by necessity, presented out of context. Legends provide the reader with a brief history of the patient's presenting complaint and a discussion of the recording.

Accurate interpretation of pediatric polysomnograms requires *complete review of the entire recording*, not just evaluation of bits and pieces. Depiction of entire polysomnograms is beyond the scope of this text. Discussions are, therefore, based on interpretation by the authors, who have had the opportunity to review the clinical history, perform a physical examination, and interpret the polysomnograms in their entirety.

Several technical comments are needed. Digital recording equipment was used to obtain all data. Nasal and oral airflow have, for the most part, been recorded by capnography and a computer algorithm was used for calculation of E_tCO_2. Because 3-second sampling time is required, there is skewing of the airflow recording by 3 seconds, making some central apnea appear as mixed apnea. Although E_tCO_2 is documented every second during a 30-second epoch, each digital representation of E_tCO_2 is an average of the prior 10 seconds of air stream sampling.

Suggested Reading

Sleep-Related Breathing Disorders

1. Anders T, Emde R, Parmalee A (eds): *A Manual of Standardized Terminology, Techniques, and Criteria for Scoring of States of Sleep and Wakefulness in Newborn Infants.* Los Angeles: UCLA Brain Information Service, 1971.
2. Carroll JL, Loughlin GM: Diagnostic criteria for obstructive sleep apnea syndrome in children. Pediatr Pulmonol 1992;14:71–74.
3. Carroll JL, Loughlin GM: Obstructive sleep apnea syndrome in infants and children: Diagnosis and management. In Ferber R, Kryger M (eds): *Principles and Practice of Sleep Medicine in the Child.* Philadelphia: W.B. Saunders, 1995, pp. 193–216.
4. Chokroverty S: Sleep and epilepsy. In Chokroverty S (ed): *Sleep Disorders Medicine.* Boston: Butterworth-Heinemann, 1994, pp. 429–455.
5. Diagnostic Classification Steering Committee, Buysse DJ (Chairman): *International Classification of Sleep Disorders, Revised: Diagnostic and Coding Manual.* Rochester, MN: 1997, pp. 195–197.
6. Fisch BJ: *Spehlmann's EEG Primer.* 2nd ed. Amsterdam: Elsevier, 1991.
7. Hillmeier AC: Gastroesophageal reflux: Diagnostic and therapeutic approaches. Pediatr Clin North Am 1996; 43:197–212.

8. Hoppenbrouwers T, Hodgman JE, Harper RM, et al: Polygraphic studies of normal infants during the first six months of life: III. Incidence of apnea and periodic breathing. Pediatrics 1977;60:418–425.
9. Kryger MH: Restrictive lung diseases. In Kryger MH, Roth T, Dement WC (eds): *Principles and Practice of Sleep Medicine*. 2nd ed. Philadelphia: W.B. Saunders, 1994, pp. 769–775.
10. Lusk RB: Congenital anomalies of the larynx. In Ballenger JJ, Snow JB (eds): *Otorhinolaryngology*. Baltimore: Williams and Wilkins, 1995, pp. 498–501.
11. Mallory GB, Fiser DH, Jackson R: Sleep associated breathing disorders in morbidly obese children and adolescents. J Pediatr 1989;115:892–897.
12. Marcus CL, Keens TG, Bautista DB, et al: Obstructive sleep apnea in children with Down syndrome. Pediatrics 1991;88:132–139.
13. Marcus CL, Curtis S, Koerner CB, et al: Evaluation of pulmonary function and polysomnography in obese children and adolescents. Pediatr Pulmonol 1996;21:176–183.
14. Martin RJ, Cicutto LC, Ballard RD: Factors related to the nocturnal worsening of asthma. Am Rev Resp Dis 1990;141:33–38.
15. Rees K, Spence DPS, Earis JE, et al: Arousal responses from apneic events during NREM sleep. Am J Respir Crit Care Med 1995;152:1016–1021.
16. Rosen CL, D'Andrea L, Haddad GG: Adult criteria for obstructive sleep apnea do not identify children with serious obstruction. Am Rev Respir Dis 1992;146: 1231–1234.
17. Rome ES, Miller MJ, Goldthwart DA, et al: Effect of sleep state on chest wall movement and gas exchange in infants with resolving bronchopulmonary dysplasia. Pediatr Pulmonol 1987;3:259–263.
18. Shannon DC, Carley DW, Kelly DH: Periodic breathing: Quantitative analysis and clinical description. Pediatr Pulmonol 1988;4:98–102.
19. Sheldon SH. *Evaluating Sleep in Infants and Children*. New York: Lippincott-Raven, 1996.
20. Sheldon SH: Sleep related enuresis. Psychiatr Clin North Am 1996;5:661–672.
21. Sheldon SH, Spire JP, Levy HB: *Pediatric Sleep Medicine*. Philadelphia: W.B. Saunders, 1992.
22. Sheldon SH, Onal E, Lilie J, et al: Sleep-related post-inspiratory upper airway obstruction in children. Sleep Res 1994;23:326.
23. Swaminathan S, Paton JY, Ward SL: Abnormal control of ventilation in adolescents with myelodysplasia. J Pediatr 1989;115:898–903.
24. Waters KA, Frobes P, Morielli A, et al: Sleep disordered breathing in children with meningomyelocele. J Pediatr 1998;132:672–681.

NREM and REM Sleep Parasomnias

1. Aldrich MS: Cardinal manifestations of sleep disorders. In Kryger MH, Roth T, Dement WC (eds): *Principles and Practice of Sleep Medicine.* Philadelphia: W.B. Saunders Co.
2. Association of Sleep Disorders Centers: *Diagnostic Classification of Sleep and Arousal Disorders.* 1st ed. Prepared by the Sleep Disorders Classification Committee, H.P. Roffwarg, Chairman. Sleep 1979;2:1–137.
3. Broughton R: Sleep disorders: Disorders of arousal? Science 1968;159:1070–1078.
4. Broughton R: Childhood sleep walking, sleep terrors and enuresis nocturna: Their pathophysiology and differentiation from nocturnal epileptic seizures. In *Sleep 1978.* Basel: S. Karger, 1980, pp. 103–111.
5. deLissovoy V: Head banging in early childhood: A study of incidence. J Pediatr 1961;58:803.
6. Diagnostic Classification Steering Committee, (MJ Thorpy Chairman): *International Classification of Sleep Disorders: Diagnostic and Coding Manual.* Rochester, Minnesota: American Sleep Disorders Association, 1990.
7. Fisher CJ, Byrne J, Edwards R, et al: A psychophysiological study of nightmares. J Am Psychoanal Assoc 1970;18:747–782.
8. Foulkes D: *Children's Dreams: Longitudinal Studies.* New York: Wiley, 1982.
9. Gastaut H, Broughton R: Paroxysmal psychological events and certain phases of sleep. Percept Motor Skills 1963; 17:362.
10. Gastaut H, Groughton RA: A clinical and polygraphic study of episodic phenomena during sleep. Rec Adv Biol Psychiat 1965;7:197.
11. Gastaut H, Broughton R: A clinical and polygraphic study of episodic phenomena during sleep. In Wortis J (ed): *Recent Advances in Biological Psychiatry.* Volume 7. New York: Plenum Press, 1965, pp. 197–223.
12. Guilleminault C: Narcolepsy and its differential diagnosis. In Guilleminault C (ed): *Sleep and its Disorders in Children.* New York: Raven Press, 1987, p. 182.
13. Kales JD, Kales A, Soldatos CR, et al: Sleep walking and night terrors related to febrile illness. Am J Psychiat 1979;136:1214–1215.
14. Kales A, Soldatos CR, Bixler EO, et al: Hereditary factors in sleepwalking and night terrors. Br J Psychiat 1980;137:111–118.
15. Kravitz H, Rosenthal, V, Teplitz Z, et al: A study of head-banging in infants and children. Dis Nerv System 1960; 21:203.
16. Lugaresi E, Cirignotta F: Hypnogenic paroxysmal dystonia: Epileptic seizure or a new syndrome? Sleep 1981; 4:129.
17. Lugaresi E, Cirignotta F: Two variants of nocturnal paroxysmal dystonia with attacks of short and long duration. In Degen R, Niedermeyer E (eds): *Epilepsy, Sleep and Sleep Deprivation.* Amsterdam: Elsevier Science Publishers, 1984, pp. 169–173.
18. Ramfjord S: Bruxism: A clinical and electromyographic study. J Am Dent Assoc 1961;62:21.
19. Sallustro MA, Atwell CW: Body rocking, head banging, and head rolling in normal children. J Pediatr 1978; 93:704–708.
20. Sheldon SH, Jacobsen J: REM-sleep motor disorder in children. J Child Neurol 1998;13:257–260.
21. Schenck C, Bundlie SR, Ettinger MG, et al: Chronic behavioral disorders of human REM sleep: A new category of parasomnia. Sleep 1986;9:293–308.
22. Schenck CH, Hurwitz TD, Mahowald MW: REM sleep behavior disorder. Am J Psychiatry 1988;145:652.
23. Schenck CH, Bundlie SR, Smith SA, et al: REM behavior disorder in a 10-year-old girl and aperiodic REM and

NREM sleep movements in an 8-year-old brother. Sleep Res 1986;15:162.

24. Schwartz SS, Gallagher RJ, Berkson G: Normal repetitive and abnormal stereotyped behavior of nonretarded infants and young mentally retarded children. Am J Ment Def 1986;90:625.

25. Yemm R: Variations in the electrical activity of the human masseter muscle occurring in association with emotional stress. Arch Oral Biol 1969;14:873–878.

Sleep in the Neurologically Challenged Child

1. American Sleep Disorders Association: *International Classification of Sleep Disorders, Revised: Diagnostic and Coding Manual.* Rochester, Minnesota: American Sleep Disorders Association, 1997, pp. 141–181.

2. Armstrong SM, Cassone VN, Chesworth MJ, et al: Synchronization of mammalian circadian rhythms by melatonin. J Neural Transm Suppl 1986;21:375–394.

3. Autret A, Laffont F, de Toffol B, et al: A syndrome of REM and non-REM sleep reduction and lateral gaze paresis after medial tegmental pontine stroke: CT scans and anatomical correlation in four patients. Arch Neurol 1988;45:1236–1242.

4. Autret A, Carrier H, Thommasi M, et al: Etude physiopathologique et neuro-pathologique d'un syndrome decortication cerebrale. Rev Neurol (Paris) 1975;131:491–504.

5. Baldy-Moulinier M, Touchon J, Besset A, et al: Sleep architecture and epileptic seizures. In Degen R, Neidermeyer E (eds): *Epilepsy, Sleep and Sleep Deprivation.* Amsterdam: Elsevier, 1984, pp. 109–118.

6. Becker PT, Thoman EB: Rapid eye movement storms in infants: Rate of occurrence at 6 months predicts mental development at 1 year. Science 1981;212:1415–1416.

7. Binnie CD, Prior PF: Electroencephalography. J Neurol Neurosurg Psychiatr 1994;57:1308–1319.

8. Bourgeois B: The relationship between sleep and epilepsy in children. Semin Pediatr Neurol 1996;3:29–35.

9. Brouillette RT, Fernbach SK, Hunt CE: Obstructive sleep apnea in infants and children. J Pediatr 1982;100:31–40.

10. Cadilhac J: Complex partial seizures and REM sleep. In Sterman MB, Shouse MN, Passouant P (eds): *Sleep and Epilepsy.* New York: Academic Press, 1982, pp. 315–324.

11. Cavallo A: The pineal gland in human beings: Relevance to pediatrics. J Pediatr 1993;123:843–851.

12. Cherubini E, Frascarelli M, Riccardi R, et al: Changes in the monosynaptic reflex during wakefulness and sleep of children with cerebral paralysis. Rivista di Neurologia 1978;48:228–241.

13. Culebras A: The neurology of sleep. Neurology 1992;42 (suppl 6):6–8.

14. Culebras A: Neuroanatomic and neurologic correlates of sleep disturbances. Neurology 1992;42(suppl 6):19–27.

15. Dahlitz M, Alvarez B, Vignau J, et al: Delayed sleep phase syndrome response to melatonin. Lancet 1991;333:1121–1124.

16. Divensky O, Ehrenberg B, Harthlen GM, et al: Epilepsy and sleep apnea syndrome. Neurology 1994;44: 2062–2064.

17. Hakamada S, Watanabe K, Hara K, et al. Body movements during sleep in full-term newborn infants. Brain Dev 1982;4:51–55.

18. Hendricks JC, Morrison AR, Mann GL: Different behaviors during paradoxical sleep without atonia depend on pontine lesion site. Brain Res 1982;239:81–105.

19. Hirsch E, Marescaux C, Maquet P, et al: Landau-Kleffner syndrome: A clinical and EEG study of five cases. Epilepsia 1990;31:756–767.

20. Jan JE, Espezel H, Appleton RE: The treatment of sleep disorders with melatonin. Dev Med Child Neurol 1994;36:97–107.

21. Jurko MF, Andy OJ, Webster CL: Disordered sleep patterns following thalamotomy. Clin Electroencephalogr 1971;2:213–217.

22. Laffont F, Autret A, Minz M, et al: Polygraphic study of nocturnal sleep in three degenerative diseases: ALS, oligoponto-cerebellar atrophy, and progressive supranuclear palsy. Wake Sleep 1979;3:17–30.

23. Lugaresi E, Cirignotta F: Hypnogenic paroxysmal dystonia: Epileptic seizure or a new syndrome? Sleep 1981;4:129–138.

24. Martin JH, Jessell TM: Development as a guide to the regional anatomy of the brain. In Kandel ER, Schwartz JH, Jessell TM: *Principles of Neural Science.* 3rd ed. New York: Elsevier, 1991, pp. 296–308.

25. Niedermeyer E: Sleep electroencephalogram in petit mal. Arch Neurol 1965;12:625–630.

26. Oksenberg A, Marks G, Farber J, et al: Effect of REM sleep deprivation during the critical period of neuroanatomical development of the cat visual system. Sleep Res 1986;15:53.

27. Rajna P, Veres J: Correlation between night sleep duration and seizure frequency in temporal lobe epilepsy. Epilepsia 1993;34:574–579.

28. Rossi GF, Colicchio G, Pola P: Interictal epileptic activity during sleep: A stereo-EEG study in patients with partial epilepsy. Electroencephalogr Clin Neurophysiol 1984;58:97–106.

29. Schenck CH, Hurwitz TD, Mahowald MW: REM sleep behavior disorder. Am J Psychiatry 1988;145:652.

30. Stahl SM, Layzer RB, Aminoff MJ, et al: Continuous cataplexy in a patient with a midbrain tumor: The limp-man syndrome. Neurology 1980;30:1115–1118.

31. Sheldon SH: *Evaluating Sleep in Infants and Children.* New York: Lippincott-Raven, 1996.

32. Sheldon SH: *Pediatric Sleep Medicine.* Philadelphia: WB Saunders Co., 1992.

33. Sheldon SH, Jacobsen JJ: REM sleep motor disorder in children. Child Neurol 1998;13:257–260.

34. Sheldon SH: Proconvulsant effects of oral melatonin in neurologically disabled children. Lancet 1998;351:1254.

35. Shibagaki M, Kiyono S, Takeuchi T: Nocturnal sleep in mentally retarded infants with cerebral palsy. Electroenceph Clin Neurophysiol 1985;61:465–471.

36. Stores G: Confusions concerning sleep disorders and epilepsys in children and adolescents. Br J Psychiatry 1991;158:1–7.

37. Tharp BR: Electrophysiological brain maturation in premature infants: An historical perspective. J Clin Neurophysiol 1990;7:302–314.

38. Ward SL, Jacobs RA, Gates EP, et al: Abnormal ventila-

tory patterns during sleep in infants with meningomyelocele. J Pediatr 1986;109:631–663.

39. Ward SL, Jacobs RA, Gates EP, et al: Abnormal ventilatory patterns during sleep in infants with myelomeningocele. J Pediatr 1986;109:631–634.

40. Ward SL, Nickerson BG, van der Hal A, et al: Absent hy-
poxic and hypercapneic arousal responses in children
with myelomeningocele and apnea. Pediatrics 1986;78:
44–50.

41. Watanabe K, Miyazaki S, Hara K, et al: Behavioral state
cycles, background EEGs and prognosis of newborns
with perinatal hypoxia. Electroenceph Clin Neurophysiol 1980;49:618–625.

42. van den Berg-Emons HJ, Saris WH, de Barbanson DC, et
al: Daily physical activity of school children with spastic
diplegia and of healthy control subjects. J Pediatr
1995;127:578–584.

Part 1

Sleep-Related Breathing Disorders

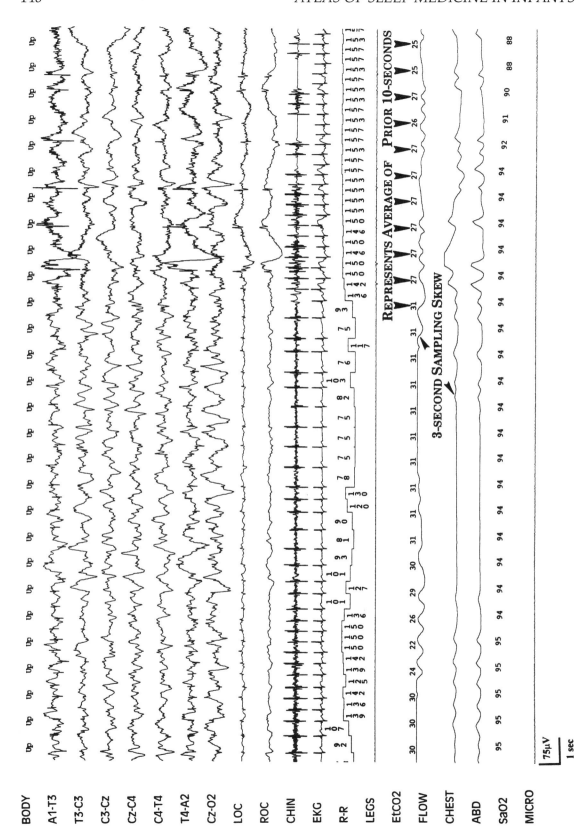

Apnea of Prematurity

Figure 38. Apnea of Prematurity

This polysomnographic segment was recorded during active sleep from a 32-week-old premature infant who was doing well in the intermediate care nursery, but was noted by nurses to have prolonged pauses in breathing associated with cardiac deceleration and pallor. Note the decreased effort and decrease in airflow lasting 15 to 20 seconds, cardiac deceleration, and mild oxygen desaturation.

Apnea of prematurity is characterized by central apnea lasting 20 seconds or longer, or by shorter central apneas associated with bradycardia, significant oxygen desaturation, and/or neurological sequelae. Prolonged spells of periodic breathing may also be present and associated with a decrease in heart rate and oxygen saturation.

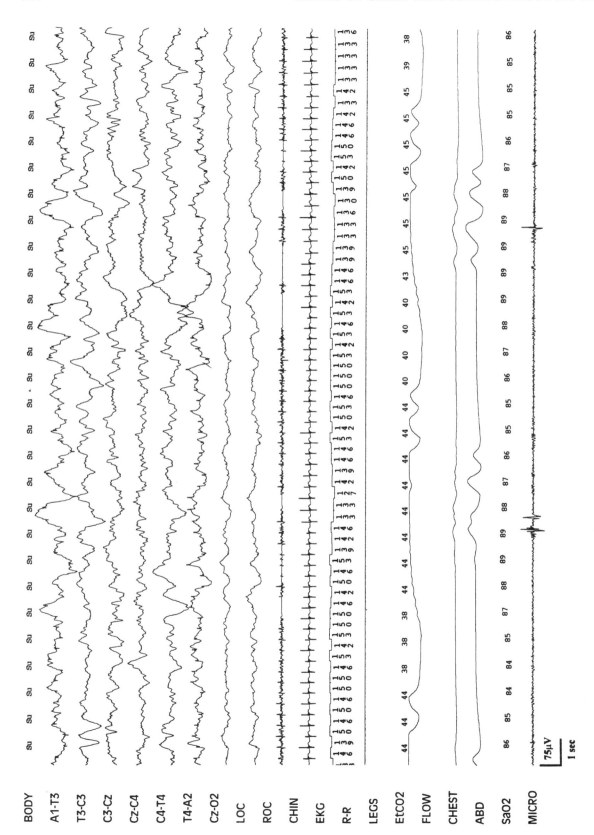

Periodic Breathing in a 2-Month-Old Male

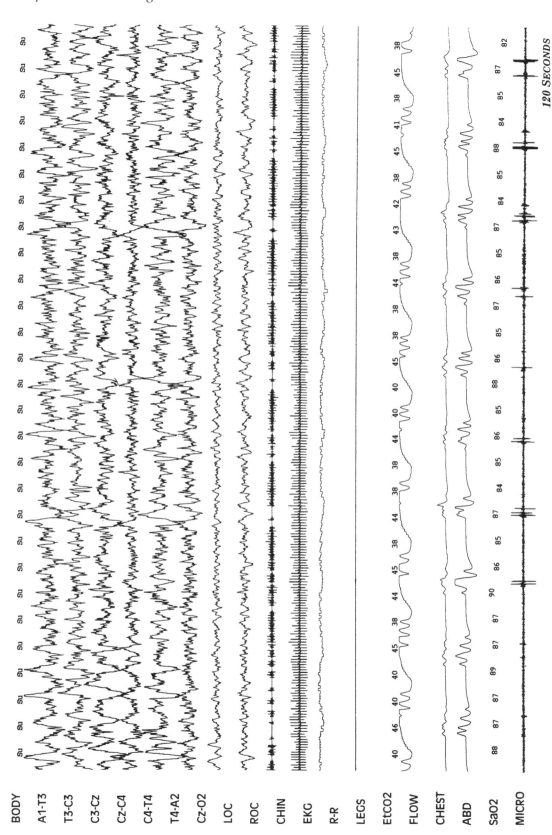

Periodic Breathing in a 2-Month-Old Male, *continued*

Figures 39a and 39b. Periodic Breathing in a 2-Month-Old Male

Figure 39a shows a 30-second polysomnographic segment, and 39b shows a 120-second polysomnographic segment obtained during quiet sleep from a 2-month-old male infant, whose parents had noted a frightening change in his breathing pattern during sleep. He was brought to the emergency department and aseptic meningitis was diagnosed. Supportive care was provided in the hospital. Note the high amplitude slow waves, predominantly tonic chin muscle tone, and absence of eye movements.

Periodic breathing was recorded throughout the infant's entire sleep period. A pattern of 7- to 10-second central respiratory pauses was identified, followed by 3 to 4 normal respiratory efforts. Note the low baseline oxygen saturation and periodicity of desaturation. This respiratory pattern of periodic breathing was likely due to the patient's central nervous system infection. Polysomnography was repeated 3 weeks after resolution of his infection, and demonstrated a normal breathing pattern with no evidence of periodic breathing.

Periodic breathing is characterized by three or more respiratory pauses of greater than 3 seconds' duration with less than 20 seconds of normal respiration between the pauses. Periodic breathing is seen primarily among preterm infants and primarily during active sleep. Although this is controversial, it may be abnormal when periodic breathing occurs in term infants for more than 5% of the total sleep time. Periodic breathing during quiet sleep may also be abnormal in the term infant and might indicate a problem in the central control of breathing, underlying pulmonary disease, or underlying cardiac disease.

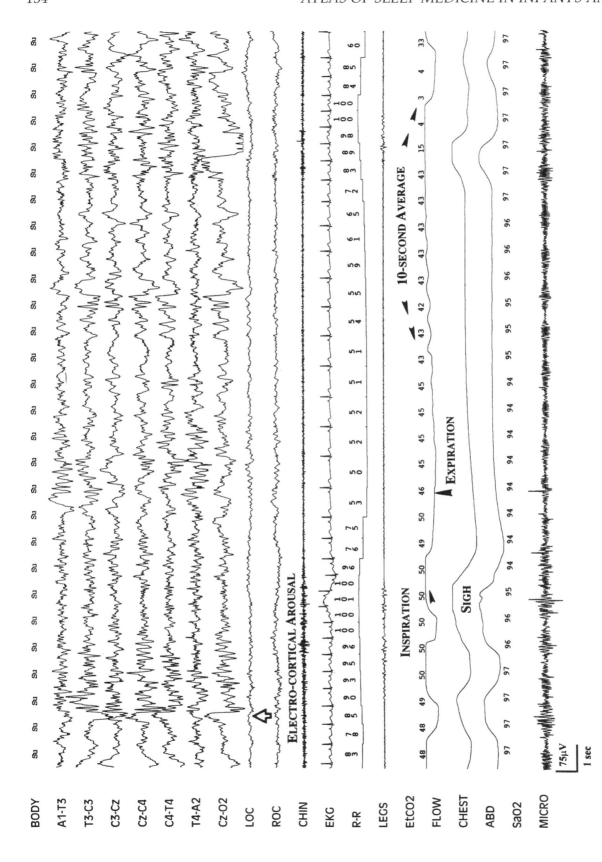

Eight-Year-Old Male with Expiratory Apnea

with progressive cardiac deceleration, with the instantaneous heart rate reaching its nadir during the last third of the apnea. Third, there is continued expiratory flow identified by continuous recording of expired carbon dioxide until the end of the pause. Finally, pulse artifact can be seen during the last 7 seconds of the pause, followed by a fall in the E_tCO_2, indicating the end of expiration prior to institution of the next inspiratory effort. Note that there is no fall in oxygen saturation during or after the respiratory pause.

Etiology, physiology, and clinical significance of expiratory apnea are unknown. Expiratory apnea may result in prolonged use of home apnea monitors. It may be a reflex-related phenomenon or may be seen as part of the syndrome of obstructive sleep apnea. Clinical correlation is typically required for the management of patients with expiratory apnea.

Figure 40. Eight-Year-Old Male with Expiratory Apnea

The polysomnographic epoch shown here was recorded from an 8-year-old male with a history of seizures. He was referred by his neurologist for evaluation of loud snoring and witnessed apnea during sleep. Sleep spindles and K complexes can be seen against a relatively low voltage, mixed frequency background, indicating stage 2 sleep.

At the beginning of the epoch, there is a brief electrocortical arousal and an augmented breath (sigh). The sigh is followed by a prolonged respiratory pause lasting about 20 seconds. The pause appears similar to a prolonged central apnea, but there are subtle differences. First, the respiratory pause is preceded by an augmented breath. Second, there is a rapid fall in the instantaneous heart rate with a slow rise in the rate as the pause in breathing continues. Pathological central apneas, on the other hand, are typically associated

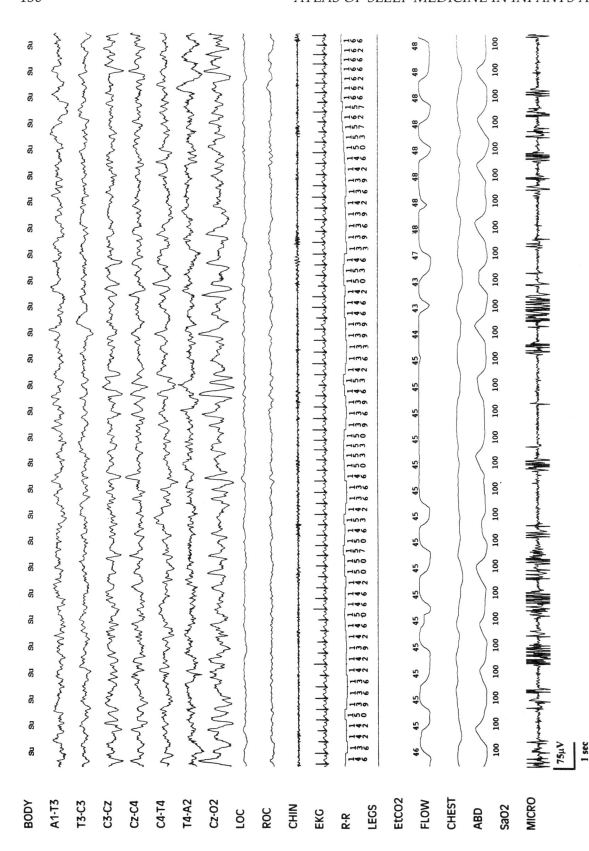

Laryngotracheomalacia Resulting in Obstructive Sleep Apnea in a 2-Month-Old Male

Figure 41a. Laryngotracheomalacia Resulting in Obstructive Sleep Apnea in a 2-Month-Old Male

Figures 41a and 41b show a recording from an infant who was referred for a history of cyanotic spells. He had been noted on physical examination to have inspiratory stridor. This polysomnographic segment was recorded during quiet sleep. Quiet sleep is identifiable by the mixed frequency, high amplitude EEG activity, the absence of eye movements, and the presence of relatively regular respiratory efforts. Note that during quiet sleep, both inspiratory and expiratory stridulous breathing was recorded.

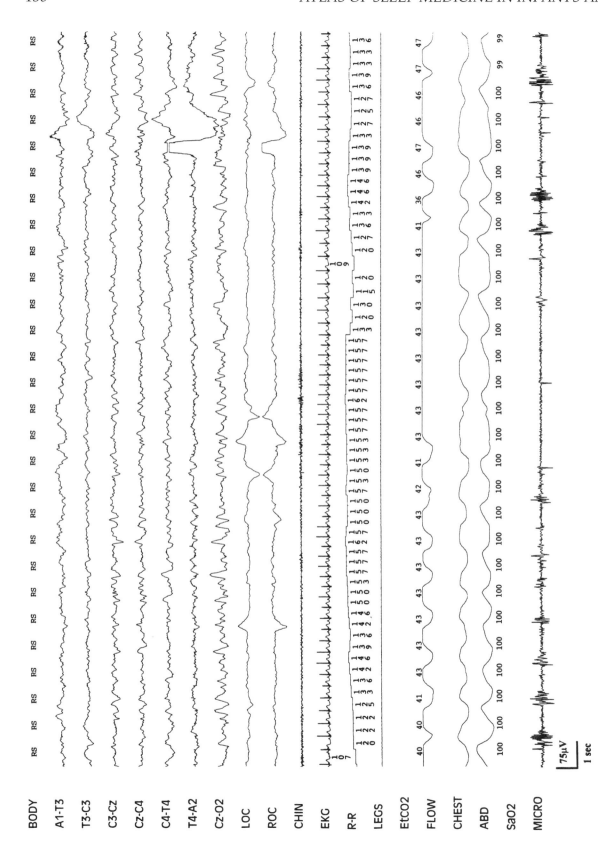

Laryngotracheomalacia Resulting in Obstructive Sleep Apnea in a 2-Month-Old Male

Figure 41b. Laryngotracheomalacia Resulting in Obstructive Sleep Apnea in a 2-Month-Old Male

This recording was obtained during active sleep. Lower amplitude, slower EEG activity, rapid eye movements, decreased chin muscle tone, and more irregular respiratory efforts are noted.

In the segments shown in Figures 41a and 41b, the patient is noted to have brief obstructive respiratory events. There is absence of airflow despite continued chest and abdominal efforts. Inspiratory sounds are noted on the sonogram before *and after* airway obstructions. Airway occlusion is associated with a transient, mild rise in E_tCO_2, but there is no associated decrease in S_pO_2.

In contrast to adult criteria for obstructive apnea, which require the absence of airflow for 10 seconds or more, even brief occlusive events are consequential in infants and children. An occlusive apnea is considered significant if there is *absence of airflow for two or more respiratory efforts*, oxygen desaturation greater than 4% from the baseline, nadir saturation below 89%, or maximum E_tCO_2 during recovery breaths greater than 53 mm Hg.

This pattern of frequent, brief respiratory obstructions associated with stridor can be consistent with, but not diagnostic of, laryngotracheomalacia. Subsequent laryngoscopy, bronchoscopy, and esophagoscopy revealed laryngotracheomalacia and inflammation extending to the middle third of the esophagus, suggesting gastroesophageal reflux.

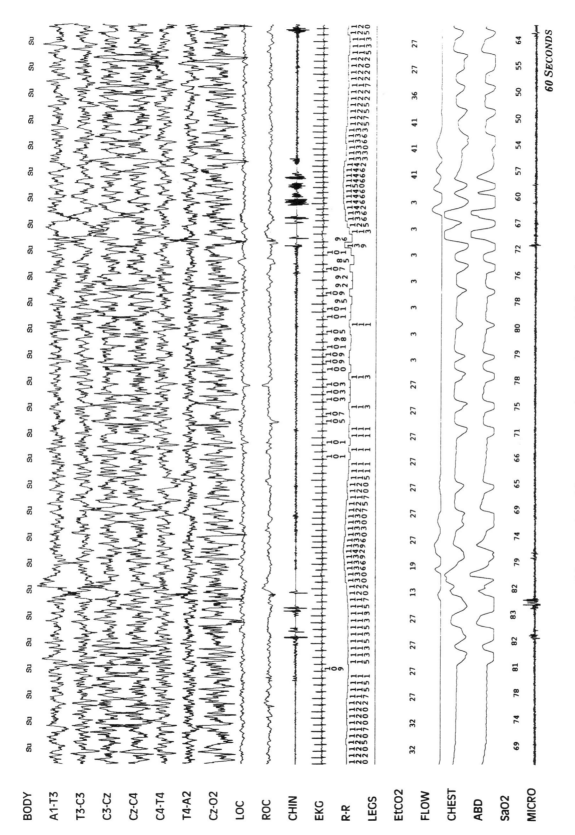

Obstructive Sleep Apnea in a 2-Year-Old Male

Figure 42. Obstructive Sleep Apnea in a 2-Year-Old Male

This 60-second polysomnographic segment was recorded from a 2-year-old male with sickle cell-thalassemia syndrome. He presented with a history of snoring and had been hospitalized frequently for vaso-occlusive crises. This epoch was obtained during REM sleep. There is a moderate voltage EEG with mixed frequency pattern, conjugate eye movements, and decreased chin tone with phasic twitches. Absence of airflow is noted for approximately 25 seconds despite continued respiratory effort in the chest and abdominal effort channels. Note the E_tCO_2 decreases to near zero. There is also mild deceleration in heart rate in the latter half of the apnea. Significant oxygen desaturation is present. The apneic episode ends with an arousal indicated by increased chin muscle tone, fast low amplitude EEG activity, and increased heart rate. Obstructive apneas were only recorded during REM sleep.

The patient was noted to have hypertrophied tonsils and adenoids and underwent tonsillectomy and adenoidectomy. Frequent vaso-occlusive crises resolved.

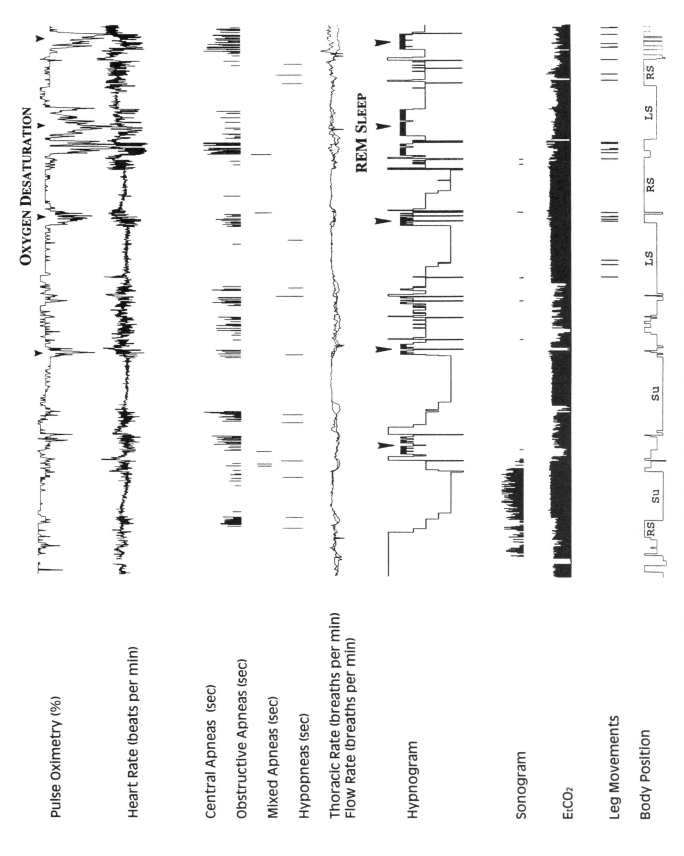

Three-Year-Old Male with Severe Obstructive Sleep Apnea

Figure 43. Three-Year-Old Male with Severe Obstructive Sleep Apnea

This hypnogram and all-night graphic summary was obtained from a 3-year-old male with hypertrophied tonsils and adenoids, chronic sinusitis, and loud snoring associated with pauses and snorts during sleep. Sleep had been described as very restless and there had been poor weight gain. Prolonged obstructive apneas were present during REM sleep, the longest lasting almost 30 seconds despite continued chest and abdominal effort. There was significant cardiac deceleration and the apneas were terminated with arousals characterized by increased EEG frequency, increased chin muscle tone, leg movements, and an audible snort. Considerable fragmentation of sleep continuity was noted.

The hypnogram and summary of this patient's recording shows oxygen desaturation and cardiac variability associated with obstructive apneas. Decreasing S_pO_2 became more evident during successive REM periods. This pattern is common among children. Early morning REM periods often exhibit the most significant occlusive events and gas exchange abnormalities. Polysomnograms that do not include several REM periods are likely to underestimate the severity of sleep-disordered breathing. Similarly, REM is rarely seen during daytime nap studies and specificity of nap studies has been shown to be quite poor.

Note the degree of fragmentation of sleep continuity. This patient had an arousal index of 26 per hour of sleep, and there were 179 state changes during the sleep period. This degree of fragmentation frequently results in increased sleepiness, which may be manifested by young children as irritability, hyperactive behavior, or falling asleep during quiet activities.

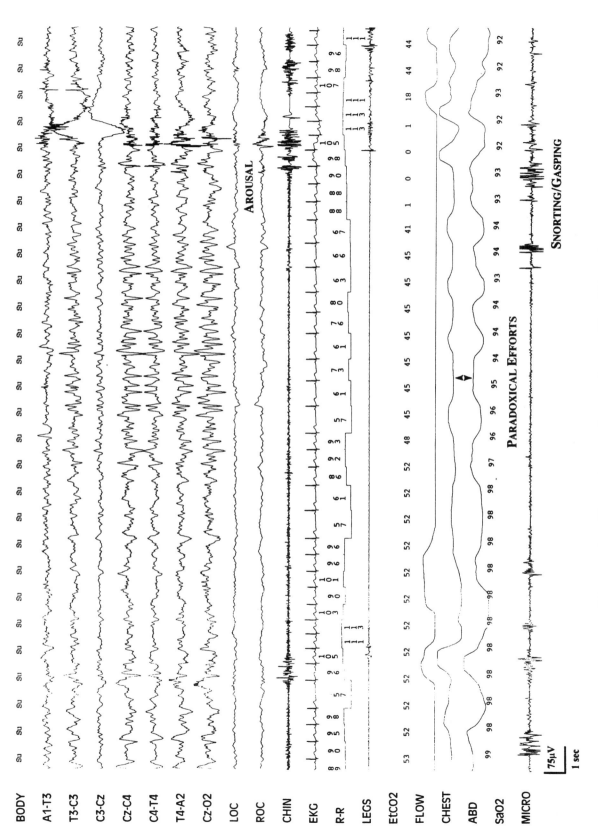

Obstructive Sleep Apnea Presenting as Head Banging

Figure 44a. Obstructive Sleep Apnea Presenting as Head Banging

The polysomnographic segments in Figures 44a and 44b were recorded from a 4-year-old male who was examined because of a complaint of recurrent episodes of head banging during the night. His history was also significant for gasping respiration.

The segment shown in Figure 44a was recorded during REM sleep. EEG background is characterized by low voltage, mixed frequency waves with bursts of notched theta activity characteristic of REM sleep. Rapid conjugate eye movements are noted and chin tone is relatively low, although increases in tone are noted during arousals near the beginning and end of the epoch. Although there is contin-

ued paradoxical effort of the chest and abdomen, there is absence of airflow for 15 seconds. E_tCO_2 falls. Since capnometry reflects the average of E_tCO_2 over the previous 10 seconds, there is a 10-second delay between the cessation of airflow and fall in E_tCO_2. Snoring is recorded sonographically before and after the apnea, but there is no snoring recorded throughout the occlusion of the upper airway. There is some slowing of the heart rate at the beginning of the apnea, suggesting an increased expiratory effort against an occluded upper airway. The apneic event is terminated with an arousal. Marked change to a waking EEG rhythm near the end of the epoch, increased chin muscle tone, increased heart rate, resumption of airflow, and snorting/gasping are noted on the sonogram.

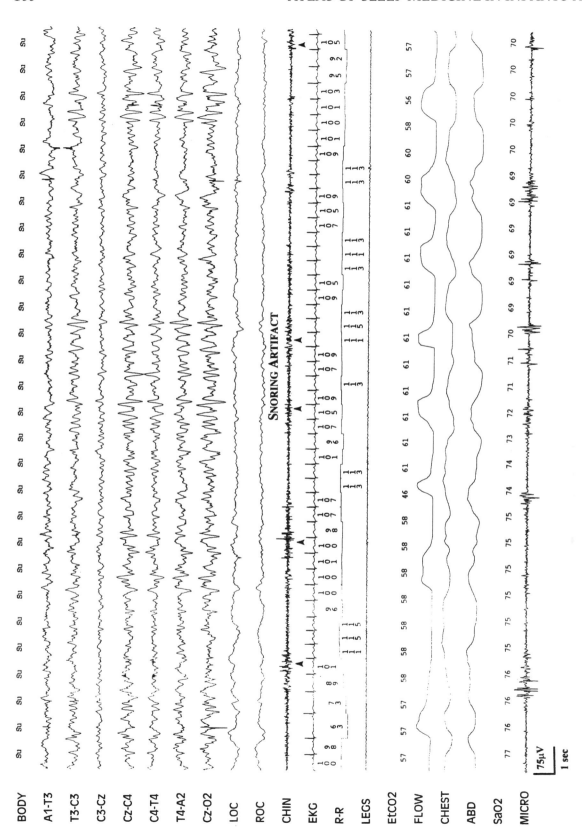

Obstructive Sleep Apnea Presenting as Head Banging

Figure 44b. Obstructive Sleep Apnea Presenting as Head Banging

Figure 44b was also recorded during REM sleep. Chin EMG reflects periodically increased vibratory tone, suggesting snoring. This is also reflected in the sonogram. E_tCO_2 is persistently elevated, with a maximum of 61 mm Hg, and significant oxygen desaturation is present. This pattern is characteristic of obstructive hypoventilation, in which there is partial, but not complete, airway obstruction. Interestingly, this child's head banging completely resolved after tonsillectomy and adenoidectomy.

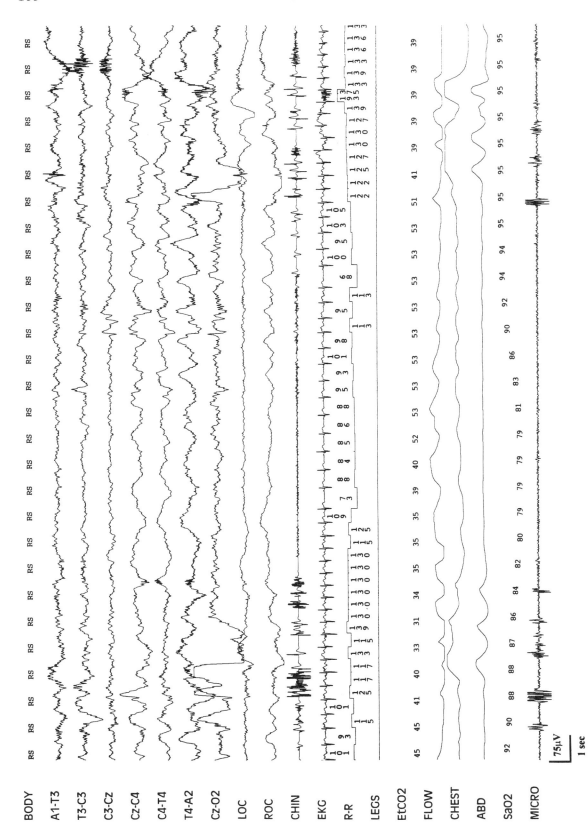

Fragmentation of Sleep Architecture by Sleep Apnea/Hypopnea

Figure 45a. Fragmentation of Sleep Architecture by Sleep Apnea/Hypopnea

The recordings in Figures 45a, 45b, and 45c were taken in an 8-year-old female with developmental delays and moderate obesity who had snoring and restless sleep despite removal of her tonsils and adenoids several years earlier. She had difficulty learning and her nasal and oral airways did not appear narrow.

This segment was recorded during stage 2 sleep and is indicative of the child's respiratory pattern during sleep. Progressive decline of airflow can be seen. This hypopnea is followed by an arousal with snoring identified on both video recording and sonography. EEG arousal, increased chin muscle tone, and increased heart rate are present. Low S_pO_2 reflects continued periodic airway occlusion from prior epochs without recovery. Elevated E_tCO_2 seen near the middle of the epoch reflects exhalation of retained carbon dioxide during arousal after the prior apnea.

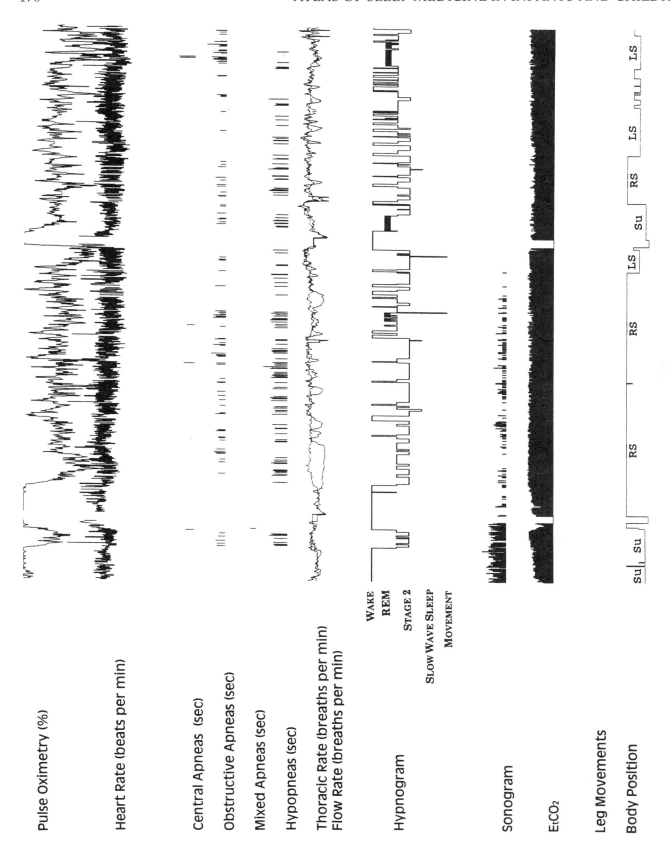

Pulse Oximetry (%)

Heart Rate (beats per min)

Central Apneas (sec)

Obstructive Apneas (sec)

Mixed Apneas (sec)

Hypopneas (sec)

Thoracic Rate (breaths per min)
Flow Rate (breaths per min)

Hypnogram

WAKE
REM
STAGE 2
SLOW WAVE SLEEP
MOVEMENT

Sonogram

EtCO₂

Leg Movements

Body Position

Fragmentation of Sleep Architecture by Sleep Apnea/Hypopnea

Figure 45b. Fragmentation of Sleep Architecture by Sleep Apnea/Hypopnea

Figure 45b represents a summary of the patient's night of sleep in the laboratory. The hypnogram reveals marked fragmentation of sleep continuity. There is no SWS and very little REM sleep recorded. There is extreme variation in oxygen saturation, and cardiac variability is due to repetitive obstructions and arousals. Numerous obstructive apneas and hypopneas are present. E_tCO_2 averages 52 mm Hg throughout the sleep period.

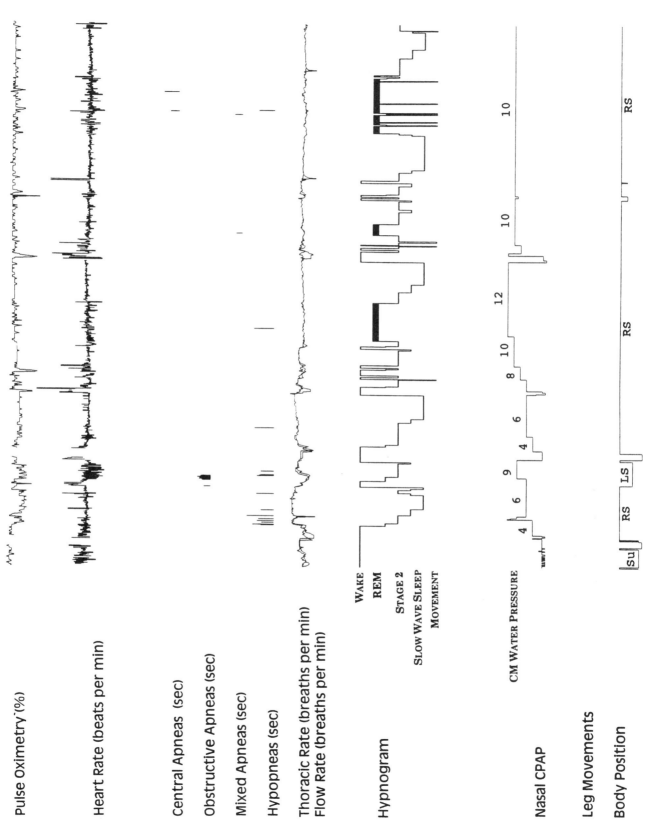

Pulse Oximetry (%)

Heart Rate (beats per min)

Central Apneas (sec)

Obstructive Apneas (sec)

Mixed Apneas (sec)

Hypopneas (sec)

Thoracic Rate (breaths per min)
Flow Rate (breaths per min)

Hypnogram

WAKE
REM
STAGE 2
SLOW WAVE SLEEP
MOVEMENT

Nasal CPAP   CM WATER PRESSURE

Leg Movements

Body Position

Fragmentation of Sleep Architecture by Sleep Apnea/Hypopnea

Figure 45c. Fragmentation of Sleep Architecture by Sleep Apnea/Hypopnea

Figure 45c shows the all-night summary recorded during the patient's night of continuous positive airway pressure (CPAP) titration. Once CPAP pressure reaches 10 cm H_2O, REM rebound occurs, SWS appears, oxygen saturation remains above 90%, and heart rate stabilizes.

This patient required a period of desensitization to the nasal CPAP mask and equipment prior to the CPAP titration. She has been able to tolerate nasal CPAP and compliance is good. She remains developmentally delayed, but her teachers have remarked that her school performance has greatly improved. Her mother has noted considerable improvement in her mood and behavior at home.

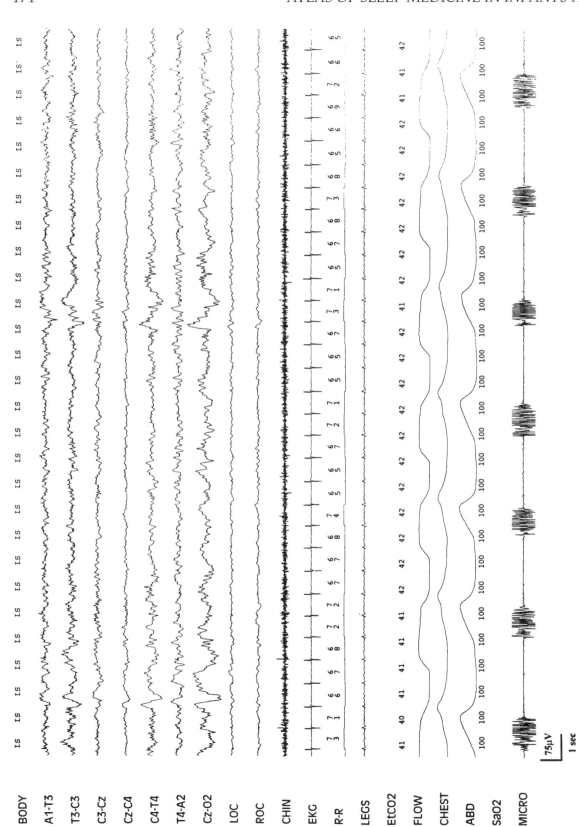

Primary Snoring in a 7-Year-Old Male

Figure 46. Primary Snoring in a 7-Year-Old Male

This polysomnographic segment was recorded from a 7-year-old male who was referred for evaluation of recurrent loud snoring. His physical examination was normal and there was no daytime symptomatology. Stage 2 sleep is seen, with a relatively low voltage, mixed frequency EEG background and clear sleep spindles. Chin muscle is tonic and heart rate shows a normal sinus variation. Respiratory rate is approximately 14 breaths per minute. There is good airflow from the nose and mouth. Snoring is recorded sonographically and is noted on the video. No other evidence of increased respiratory work from high upper airway resistance (such as paradoxical respiratory efforts), increased E_tCO_2, oxygen desaturation, frequent arousals, or architectural changes are noted. In the absence of diurnal symptoms, this polysomnogram is consistent with primary snoring.

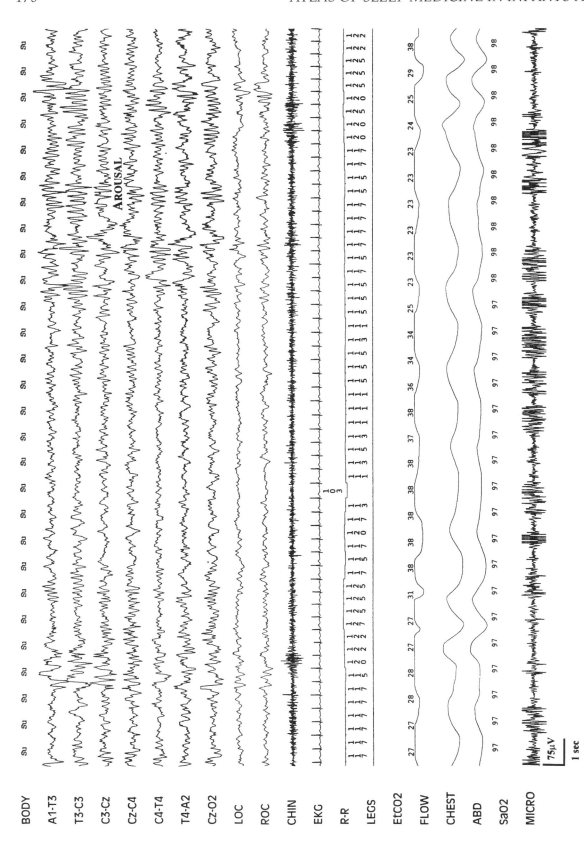

Obstructive Sleep Apnea in a 17-Month-Old Male

Figure 47a. Obstructive Sleep Apnea in a 17-Month-Old Male

This 17-month-old male was hospitalized because of gastroesophageal reflux and frequent nocturnal awakenings. He was noted to have adeno-tonsillar hypertrophy. Loud snoring was noted by his nurses. This polysomnographic segment was recorded during stage 2 sleep. There is relatively high chin muscle tone, mixed amplitude EEG waves, and no evidence of eye movements. Periodic increasing chest and abdominal effort, decreased airflow, and decreased E_tCO_2 suggest recurrent obstructive hypopneas. Snoring is also present. This subtle occlusion of the upper airway is terminated by an arousal, with increased EEG frequency, increased chin tone, and increased airflow. There is no significant change in S_pO_2.

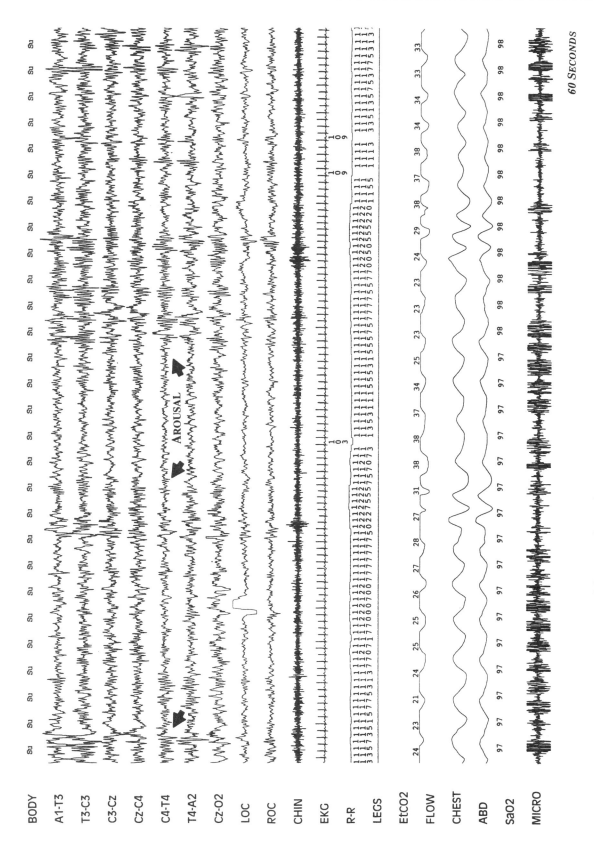

Obstructive Sleep Apnea in a 17-Month-Old Male

uration associated with the partial obstructive events, a great number of arousals were present, resulting in severe fragmentation of the continuity of sleep. This patient had markedly reduced SWS and poor sleep efficiency. Tonsillectomy and adenoidectomy led to much improved sleep quality. A follow-up polysomnogram 4 weeks after the surgery was normal.

Figure 47b. Obstructive Sleep Apnea in a 17-Month-Old Male

This figure shows a *60-second* epoch of the same phenomenon seen in Figure 47a. Recurrent nature of the subtle hypopneas is more readily seen. Periodic waxing and waning of the patient's snoring can also be seen. Although this patient did not have significant oxygen desat-

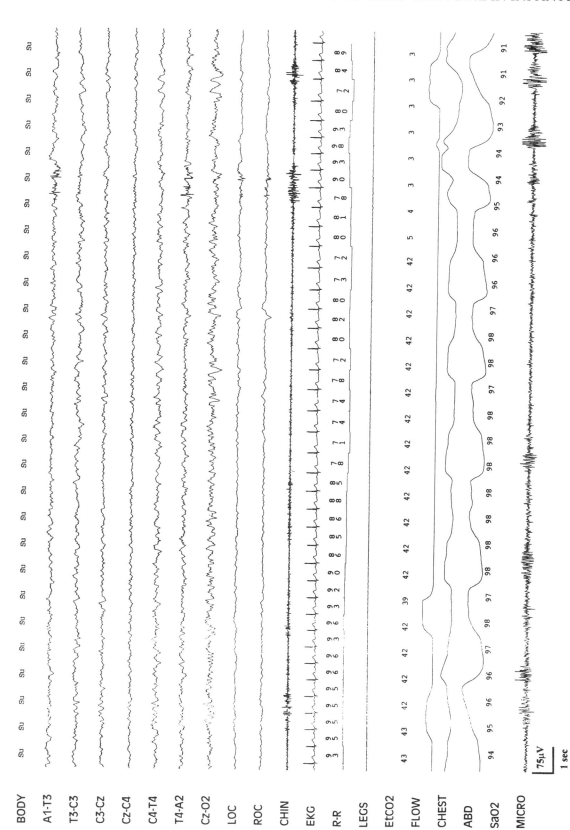

Thirteen-Year-Old Male with Obstructive Sleep Apnea and Enuresis

Figure 48. Thirteen-Year-Old Male with Obstructive Sleep Apnea and Enuresis

A 13-year-old male presented to the Sleep Medicine Center receiving a diagnosis of primary sleep-related enuresis by his primary care practitioner. Multiple behavioral and medical interventions failed to solve this patient's problem bed wetting. His mother noted that he snored loudly when sleeping and that the snoring was associated with pauses and snorts. He did not wake at night. He was somewhat hyperactive during the day, was doing poorly in school, was considered lazy by his teachers, and regularly took 3-hour naps on weekends despite sleeping approximately 9 hours per night. Moderate tonsillar hypertrophy and retrognathia was present on physical examination.

This polysomnographic segment was recorded during REM sleep in the 13-year-old patient. Background EEG reveals a relatively low voltage, mixed frequency pattern (predominantly in the theta range), similar to that seen in adult REM sleep. Decreased chin muscle tone is present. Ongoing paradoxical respiratory efforts can be seen in the chest and abdominal recording. Airflow is absent for approximately 18 seconds. There is very mild cardiac deceleration and a mild fall in oxygen saturation. This obstructive apnea is terminated by a brief arousal. The patient was then referred for an adeno-tonsillectomy. Complete resolution of his enuresis occurred 2 weeks after surgery. School performance improved and habitual napping on weekends was abandoned.

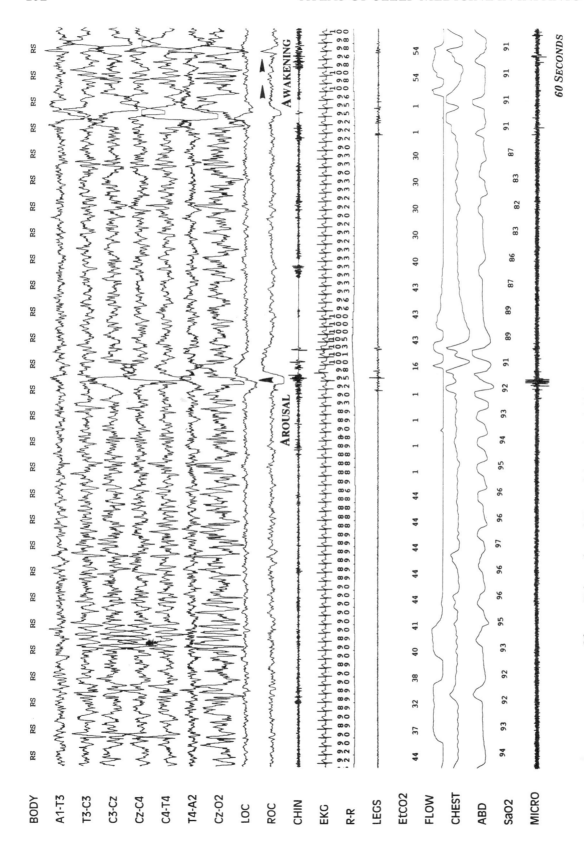

Sleep-Disordered Breathing in Children with Down Syndrome

Figure 49a. Sleep-Disordered Breathing in Children with Down Syndrome

Children with Down syndrome (trisomy 21) are at high risk for sleep-disordered breathing because of their relatively small airway and low muscle tone. Obstructive sleep apnea can persist in this population of patients even after adeno-tonsillectomy.

Figure 49a is a *60-second* polysomnographic segment recorded from a 4-year-old with Down syndrome, loud snoring, restless sleep, and frequent nocturnal awakenings. Note the two obstructive apneas associated with a fall in E_tCO_2 and significant oxygen desaturation. The first apnea is terminated with increased respiratory effort, as indicated by increased chin muscle tone. It is followed by three breaths during which there is good airflow. This obstructive apnea is immediately followed by another occlusive event, again terminated by an arousal and associated with a snorting sound. This second occlusive event results in an arousal and full awakening. This pattern of upper airway obstruction was seen during each episode of REM sleep.

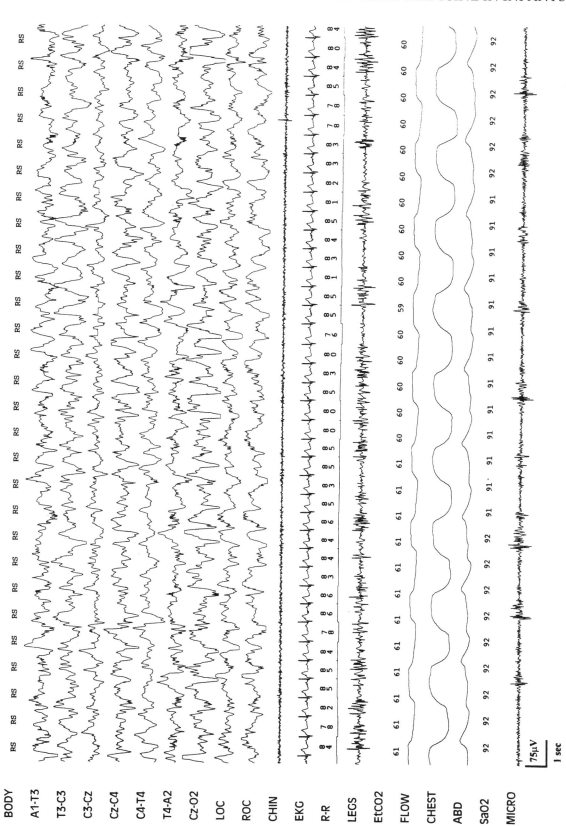

Sleep-Disordered Breathing in Children with Down Syndrome

Figure 49b. Sleep-Disordered Breathing in Children with Down Syndrome

This figure shows a 30-second polysomnogram segment recorded from a 10-year-old female with Down syndrome, morbid obesity, loud snoring, and restless sleep. She had undergone adeno-tonsillectomy approximately 1 year prior to this sleep study. SWS with characteristic delta waves dominating the EEG is demonstrated. No apnea is noted. Snoring, paradoxical respiratory effort, low baseline oxygen saturation, and persistently elevated E_tCO_2 are clearly present. This pattern of *obstructive hypoventilation* can clinically be associated with as much daytime impairment of attention and mood as overt apnea, and can result in similar physiological morbidity.

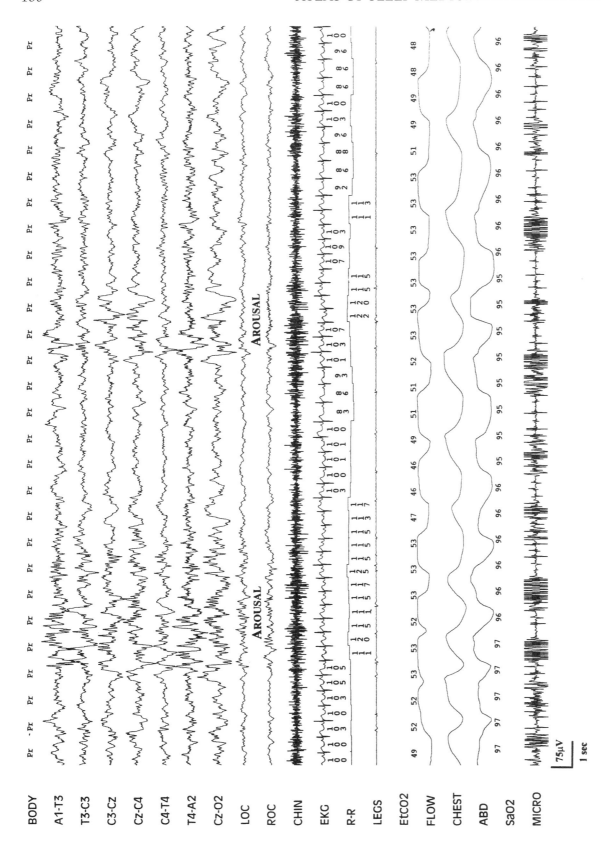

Obstructive Hypoventilation in a 4-Year-Old Male

Figure 50. Obstructive Hypoventilation in a 4-Year-Old Male

This polysomnographic segment was recorded from a 4-year-old who was referred for evaluation of snoring, gasping during sleep, and restless sleep. He had undergone polysomnography for snoring 2 years previously, but the study at that time revealed only rare REM-related obstructions and no significant sleep-disordered breathing.

State 2 sleep is depicted on this epoch. Snoring is noted sonographically. Neither apneas nor hypopneas can be seen. However, E_tCO_2 is somewhat elevated. S_pO_2 is also slightly lower than would be expected for a child this age. Two electrocortical arousals are noted in this 30-second epoch. Arousals are associated with in-

creased heart rate, increased chin muscle tone, and K complexes followed by brief periods of fast EEG activity without state change. This patient's sleep was extremely fragmented by multiple arousals. His arousal index was over 40 per hour of sleep.

Whereas discrete obstructive hypopneas are seen in the adult patient, obstructive hypoventilation may be a more common presentation of similar pathophysiological phenomena in children. Obstructive hypoventilation occurs when the maximum E_tCO_2 is greater than 53 mm Hg, when E_tCO_2 remains greater than or equal to 47 mm Hg for more than 60% of the total sleep time, or when associated oxygen desaturation falls below 89%.

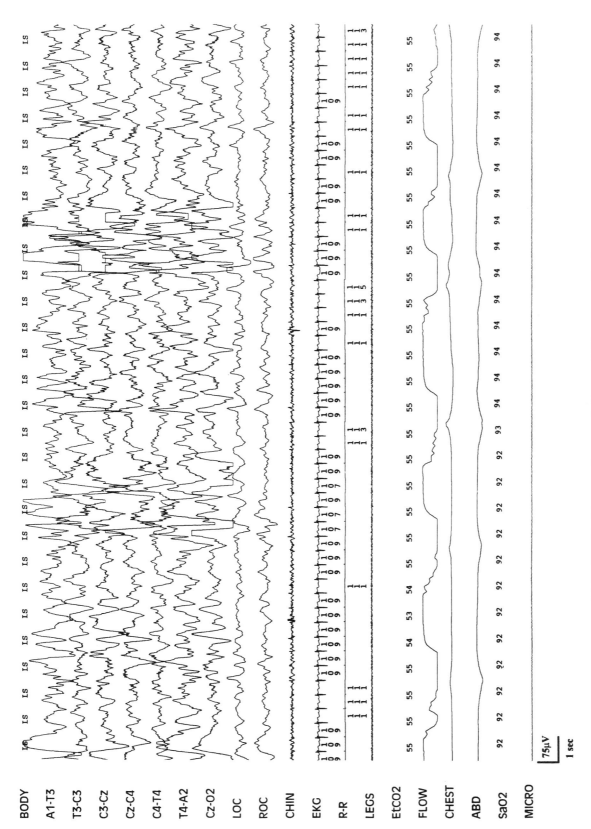

Chiari II Malformation and Central Hypoventilation

Figure 51a. Chiari II Malformation and Central Hypoventilation

The two polysomnographic segments shown in Figures 51a and 51b were recorded from a 7-year-old female with Chiari II malformation. She was referred for a polysomnogram to evaluate her respiratory status prior to a neuro-surgical procedure. A tracheotomy tube had previously been inserted because of severe obstructive sleep apnea syndrome, but she had not required ventilatory support.

The segment shown in this figure was recorded during SWS. There is a preponderance of high voltage slow waves seen on EEG. Respiratory rate is 12 breaths per minute. Oxygen saturation remains above 92%, but E_tCO_2 is quite elevated.

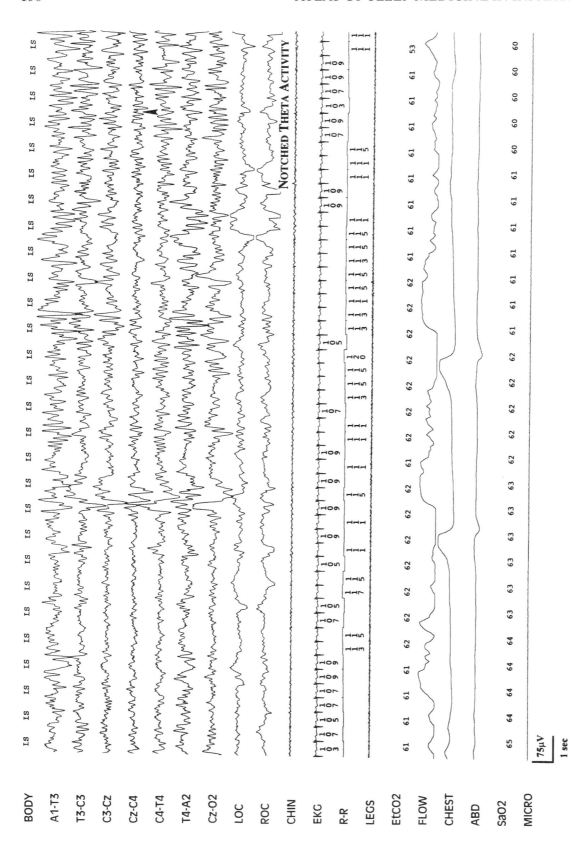

Chiari II Malformation and Central Hypoventilation

piratory effort has decreased and respiratory rate has slowed to six breaths per minute. E_tCO_2 is markedly elevated and S_pO_2 falls to a low of 60%. Decreased chemosensitivity to both hypercapnea and hypoxia is demonstrated in this patient. She responded very well to mechanical ventilatory support during sleep.

Figure 51b. Chiari II Malformation and Central Hypoventilation

    This polysomnographic segment was recorded from the same patient during REM sleep. There is a relatively moderate voltage, mixed frequency EEG background with notched theta activity. Central res-

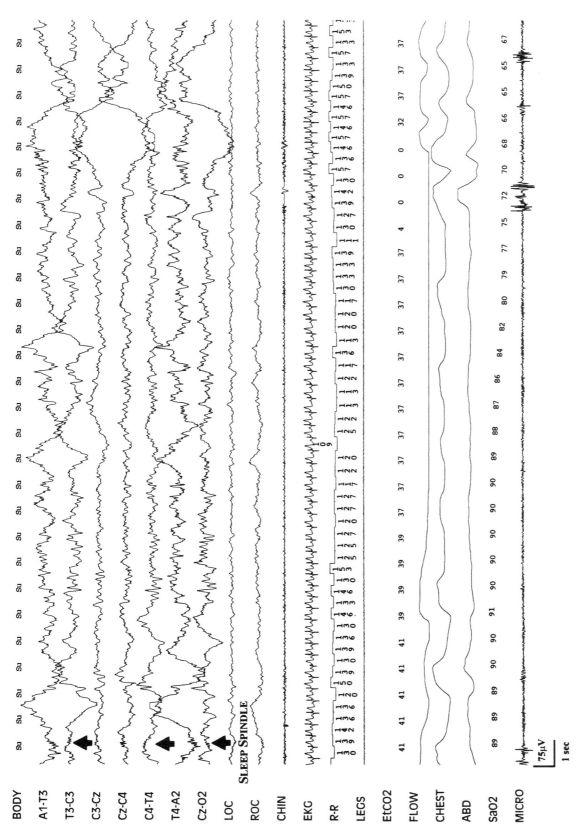

Restrictive and Obstructive Airway Disease

Figure 52a. Restrictive and Obstructive Airway Disease

The polysomnographic segments in Figures 52a and 52b were recorded from a 5-year-old female with a thoracic meningomyelocele, a ventriculo-peritoneal shunt, and severe kyphoscoliosis. There were no specific sleep-related complaints. This study was done as part of a comprehensive preoperative evaluation for correction of her kyphoscoliosis.

This polysomnographic segment was recorded during stage 2 sleep. There is a relatively low voltage, mixed frequency EEG background. Low voltage sleep spindles can be seen. Chin muscle is tonic. EKG reveals a sinus tachycardia with normal respiratory variation. Respiratory rate is elevated at 26 breaths per minute. A 16-second obstructive apnea is present and is associated with significant oxygen desaturation. E_tCO_2 remains within a normal range of 35 to 40 mm Hg. Relatively rapid, shallow breathing associated with restrictive skeletal component was present. Increased ventilation of dead space resulted in apparently normal E_tCO_2.

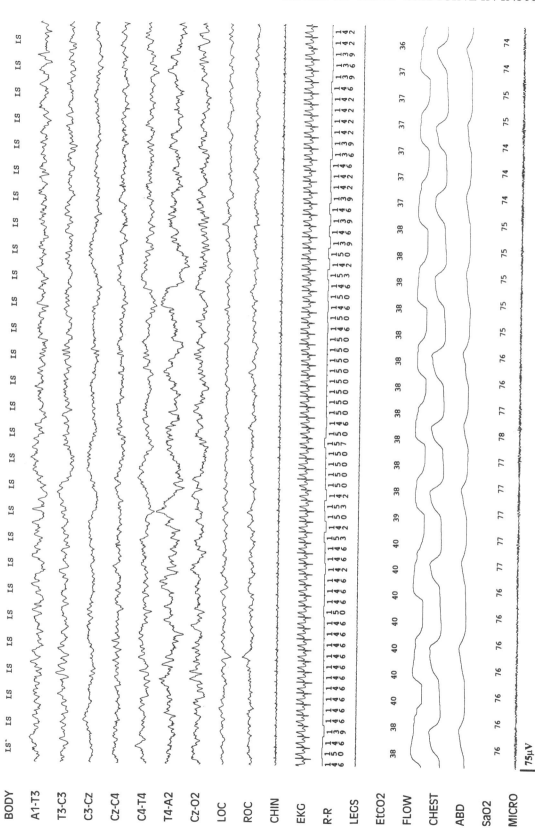

Restrictive and Obstructive Airway Disease

Figure 52b. Restrictive and Obstructive Airway Disease

This polysomnographic segment was recorded during REM sleep. Although no clear obstructive apneas or hypopneas are present, oxygen saturation baseline is significantly low. Because a normal decrease in skeletal muscle tone associated with REM sleep is present, this patient is unable to recruit accessory muscles of respiration. REM sleep hypotonia, in addition to the chest wall restriction due to deformity, resulted in a decreased tidal volume, and minute ventilation during sleep is also decreased. Respiratory rate drops from 26 breaths per minute to 20 breaths per minute. E_tCO_2 continues to appear normal. However, simultaneous measurement of transcutaneous CO_2 (T_cPCO_2) revealed 65 mm Hg, confirming alveolar hypoventilation, most likely due to a combination of airway obstruction and chest wall restriction.

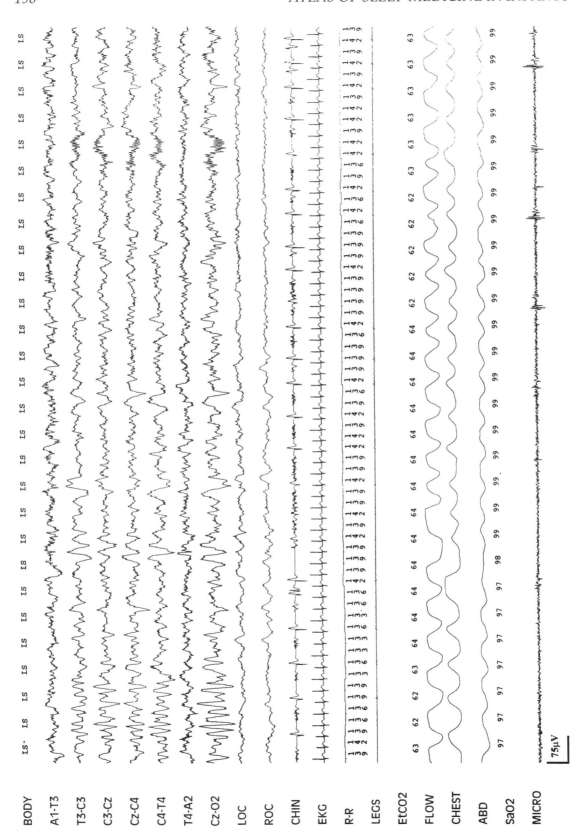

Alveolar Hypoventilation Due to Chronic Lung Disease

Figure 53. Alveolar Hypoventilation Due to Chronic Lung Disease

This polysomnographic segment was recorded from a 2-year-old male with a history of extreme prematurity, severe bronchopulmonary dysplasia, and continuous supplemental oxygen requirement. This study was performed with supplemental oxygen at a flow rate of 1.5 L/min. Sleep spindles and K complexes can be identified in this 30-second epoch of stage 2 sleep. Respiratory rate is significantly elevated at approximately 48 breaths per minute. There is no snoring, heart rate is regular, and airflow appears normal. Oxygen saturation remains greater than 95% with supplemental oxygen. E_tCO_2 is elevated, suggesting alveolar hypoventilation. Chest and abdominal efforts appear normal. This patient's carbon dioxide retention is most likely due to a diffusion defect secondary to his underlying lung disease.

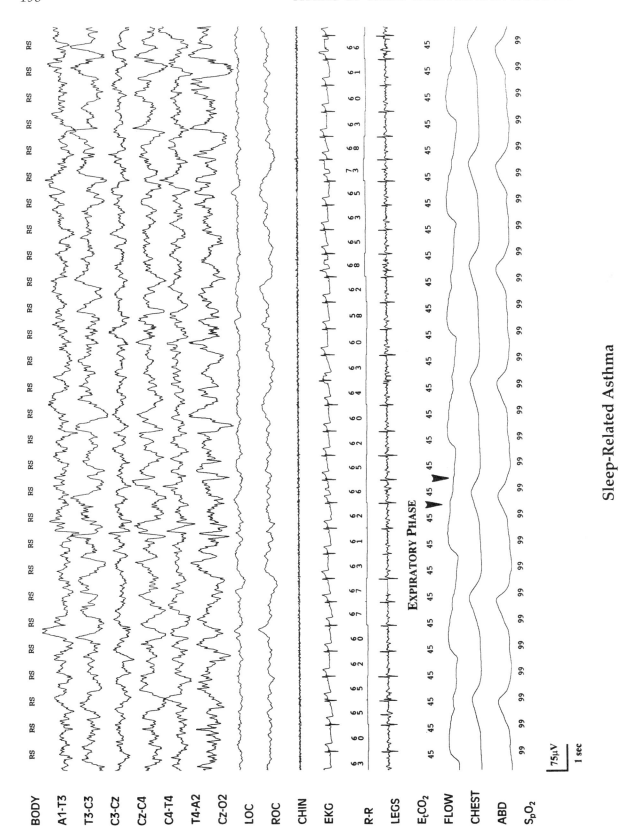

Sleep-Related Asthma

Figure 54. Sleep-Related Asthma

This 30-second polysomnographic segment was recorded from a 10-year-old male with a history of reactive airways disease, who was referred for possible sleep-disordered breathing. The patient is in early SWS. More than 20% of the epoch consists of high voltage activity with a frequency of less than 2 Hz. Chin muscle is tonic, there are no rapid eye movements, and respiratory effort is very regular.

Respiratory rate is 14 breaths per minute. Oxygen saturation is normal and airflow appears normal. E_tCO_2 is normal. However, there is a very prolonged expiratory phase of the patient's respiratory cycle. In the absence of upper airway obstruction, lower airway obstruction is suggested as a source of this patient's sleep-disordered breathing. Wheezing was confirmed by chest auscultation and it resolved after albuterol nebulization was administered.

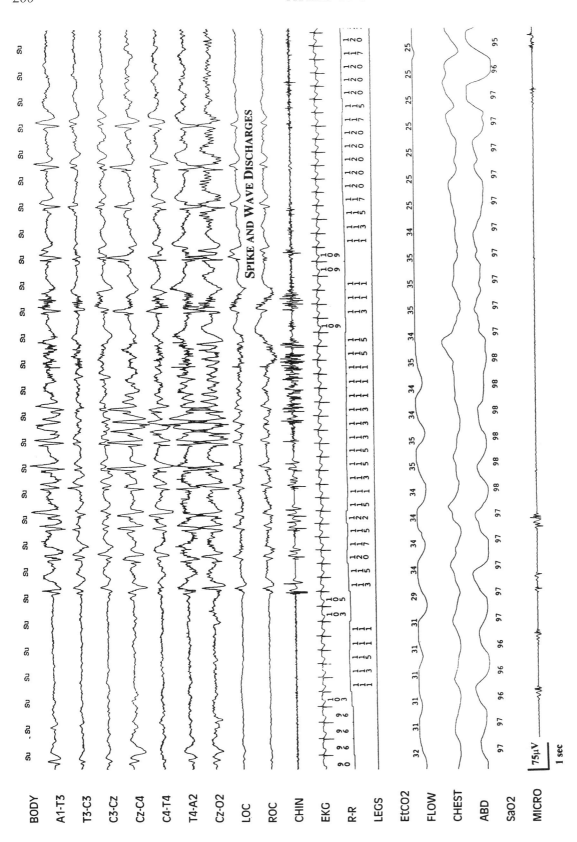

Apnea Associated with Epileptiform Activity

Figure 55. Apnea Associated with Epileptiform Activity

This 30-second polysomnogram segment was obtained from a 12-year-old male with severe mental retardation, cerebral palsy, and a history of seizures. During a prior hospitalization, he was noted to experience oxygen desaturations while sleeping. A polysomnogram was ordered.

Background EEG activity consists of very low voltage wave forms interrupted by a burst of hypersynchronous high voltage slow wave and spike/wave complexes. Although there is no increase in muscle activity during this episode, heart rate increases from the baseline. A series of five spike and wave discharges followed by EEG attenuation is accompanied by an obstructive apnea associated with mild oxygen desaturation. Paroxysmal episodes of sleep-disordered breathing (obstructive and/or central apneas) may be the only clinical manifestation of seizure activity during sleep. Generalized sleep-related seizures may or may not be associated with clinical manifestations and electrical seizure activity is more accurately termed epileptiform, rather than epileptic.

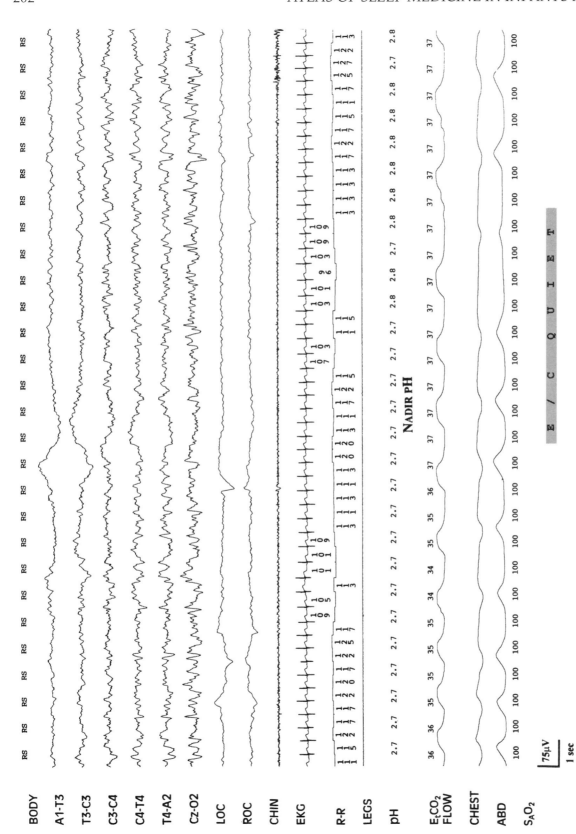

Sleep-Related Gastroesophageal Reflux

Figure 56a. Sleep-Related Gastroesophageal Reflux

The polysomnogram segments shown in Figures 56a and 56b were recorded from two different 2-month-old infants. Both were referred for evaluation of ALTEs. Polysomnography with simultaneous pH monitoring was performed as part of the comprehensive work-up. Figure 56a demonstrates 30 seconds of active sleep. There is mod-

erate voltage continuous EEG activity, conjugate eye movements, and low chin muscle tone. Sustained eye closure is present. Normal respiratory instability associated with active sleep is present. Esophageal pH monitor reveals an episode of reflux with the pH falling to a nadir of 2.7. The patient is quiet and no apneas are associated with this episode of reflux.

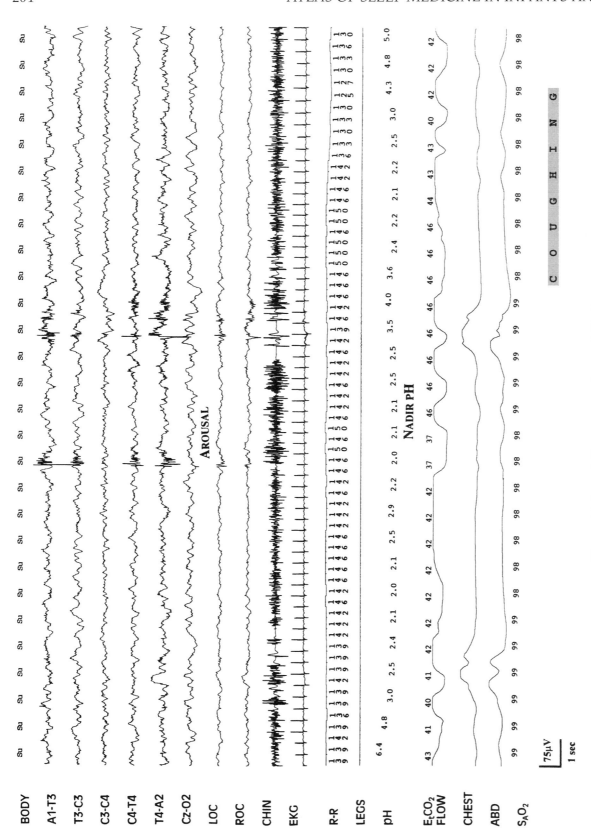

Sleep-Related Gastroesophageal Reflux

Figure 56b. Sleep-Related Gastroesophageal Reflux

Figure 56b shows a 30-second epoch recorded from a 2-month-old infant during indeterminate sleep. In comparison to Figure 56a, this epoch reveals a precipitous drop in pH from 6.4 to a low of 2.1, indicating reflux. There is an concurrent abrupt arousal, exemplified by change in EEG amplitude and frequency, increase in heart rate, increase in muscle tone, gross motor movement, *and coughing* documented by the technician. Two episodes of cessation of airflow can be seen, each lasting approximately 7 seconds. Brief apneas during wakefulness may be related to vocalizations, however, they may also be related to brief episodes of laryngospasm in an attempt to protect the airway from aspiration of gastric contents refluxed into the pharynx.

Part 2

Non-REM
Sleep-Related Parasomnias

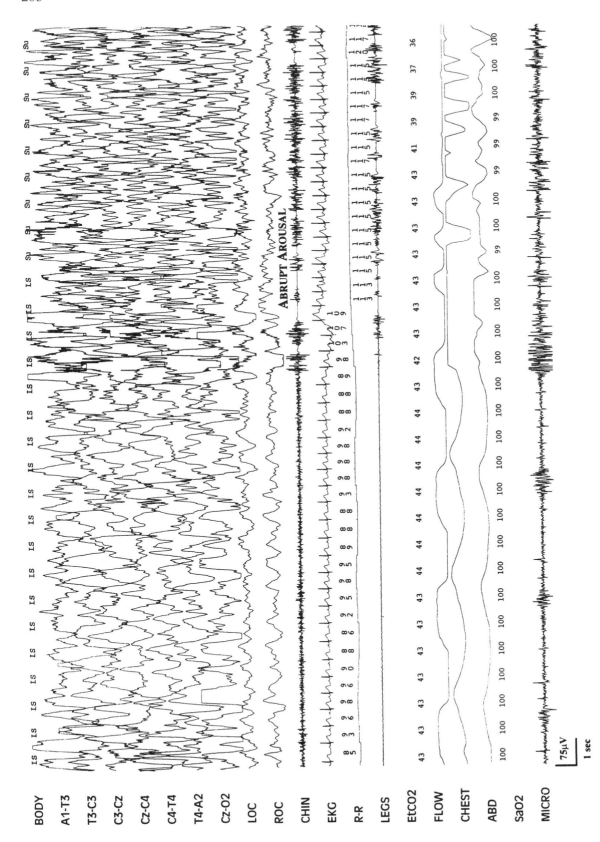

Nonspecific Features of NREM Partial Arousal Disorders

Figure 57a. Nonspecific Features of NREM Partial Arousal Disorders

NREM partial arousal disorders are fairly common during childhood and may be characterized by a variety of symptoms and motor manifestations. These can range from quietly sitting up in bed during sleep to frantic movements, displacement from bed, and complex automatisms. Multiple episodes can take place during a single sleep period. Severe injury can occur and spells can be potentially fatal, given the severity of agitation and environmental hazards.

Overt clinical manifestations are often absent during laboratory testing, even in patients who experience multiple spells during the night. Several nonspecific findings may occur, however, and may be consistent with these NREM motor parasomnias. These findings include theta delta intrusion into SWS resulting in a *theta-delta sleep* pattern, intermittent *hypersynchronous* delta EEG activity, and frequent *brief electrocortical arousals in SWS without state change.* Polysomnographic characteristics are, of course, age dependent. The younger the child, the less consistently clinical manifestations are associated with these findings, suggesting a maturational etiology. *Although these very nonspecific findings are not diagnostic of NREM partial arousal motor parasomnias, if assessed along with a characteristic history, they seem to be consistent with this presumed maturational problem.*

These polysomnographic epochs were recorded from a 5-year-old male with a history of agitated sleep walking. Spells occurred about five to seven times per week. The child was injured on two separate occasions: he sustained a lip laceration after falling over furniture, and multiple lacerations after running through a sliding glass door. There was amnesia for all events.

The segment in Figure 57a was recorded during SWS and demonstrates an abrupt partial arousal. Note the sudden appearance of muscle and movement artifact, increase in chin muscle tone, increase in heart rate, and increase in respiratory rate. EEG background activity during the movements is approximately 1 Hz and there is no clear state change. Video recording of the spell documented the patient sitting up, shouting incoherently, and pulling at the bed linen.

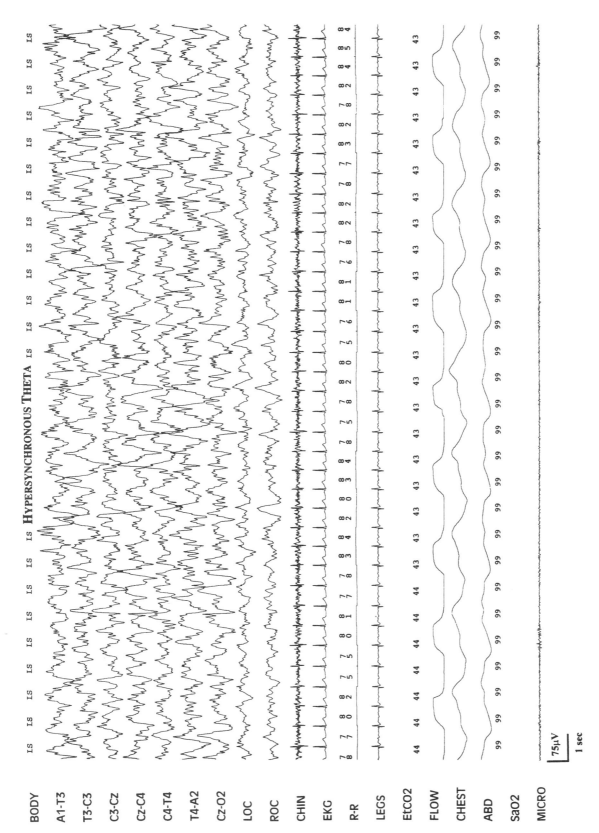

Nonspecific Features of NREM Partial Arousal Disorders

Figure 57b. Nonspecific Features of NREM Partial Arousal Disorders

This figure demonstrates intrusion of hypersynchronous theta activity into SWS resulting in a "theta-delta" sleep pattern. It is not yet known whether this phenomenon is a pediatric analog to "alpha-delta" sleep in adults.

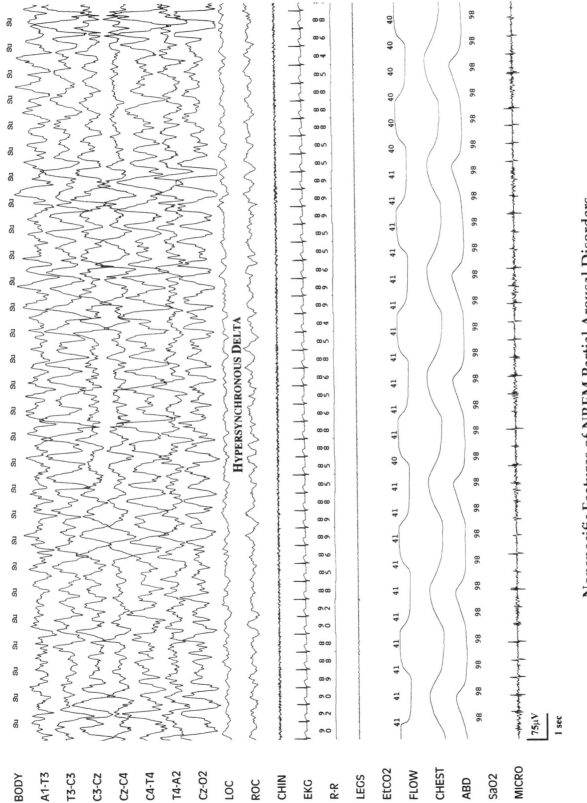

Nonspecific Features of NREM Partial Arousal Disorders

Figure 57c. Nonspecific Features of NREM Partial Arousal Disorders

This figure demonstrates a period of hypersynchronous delta activity during SWS.

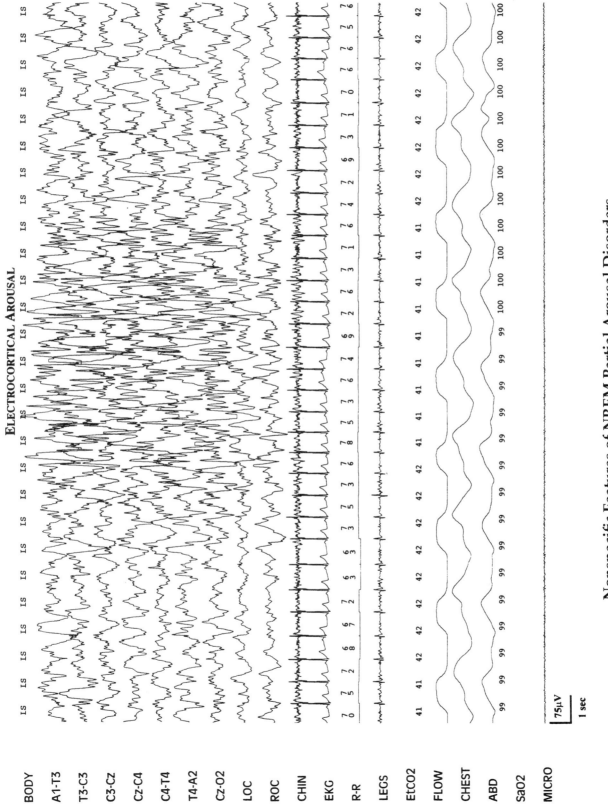

Nonspecific Features of NREM Partial Arousal Disorders

Figure 57d. Nonspecific Features of NREM Partial Arousal Disorders

The polysomnographic segment in this figure demonstrates brief electrocortical arousals during SWS unaccompanied by state change.

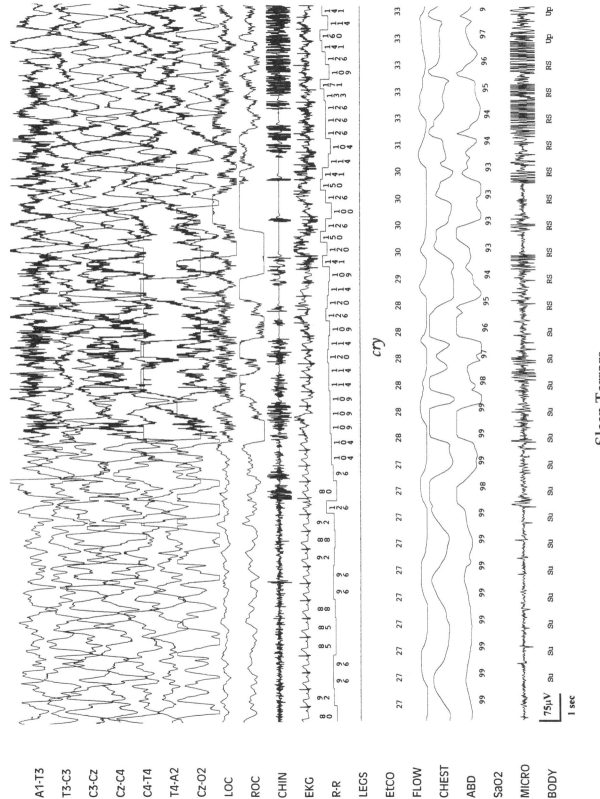

Sleep Terrors

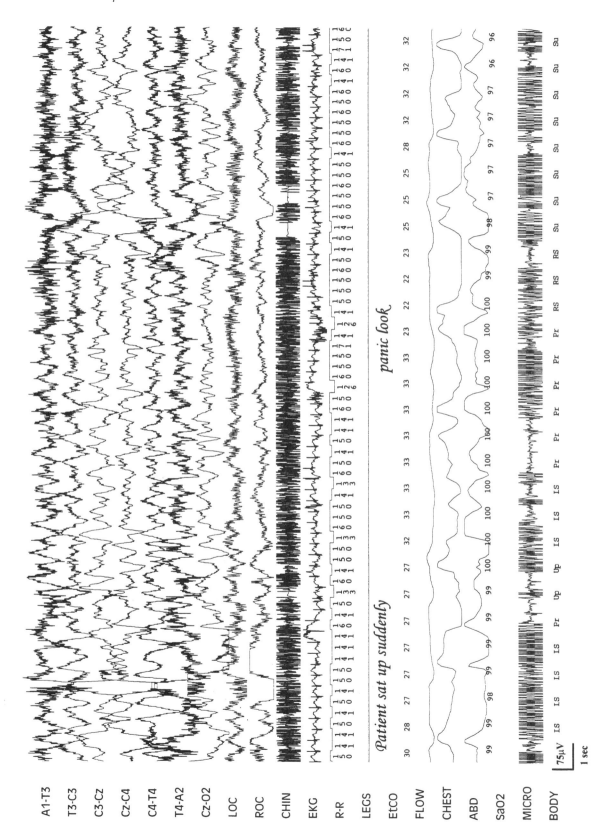

Sleep Terrors, *continued*

Figures 58a and 58b. Sleep Terrors

The polysomnogram segments shown in Figures 58a and 58b have been recorded from a 21/4-year-old male who presented to the Pediatric Sleep Medicine Clinic with a history of abrupt onset of screaming as if terrified, occurring only during sleep. The boy's parents reported that he would suddenly sit up in bed, yelling uncontrollably, and that he was unresponsive to parental interventions. Attempts to comfort him usually resulted in worsening of symptoms. During spells, he was diaphoretic, tachypneic, tachycardic, and produced unintelligible vocalizations. Episodes would begin approximately 1 to 2 hours after sleep onset, last about 5 to 10 minutes, then resolve quickly and spontaneously. Spells occurred several times per night. No injuries were reported, but there was very significant disruption of sleep of the entire family. This clinical history was consistent with sleep terrors. Polysomnographic evidence is typically nonspecific, and is diagnostic only if the child has a characteristic spell documented in the laboratory.

Figure 58a was recorded during SWS. Note the abrupt and sudden arousal with movement/muscle artifact, obscuring the majority of the EEG. Slow, 0.1-Hz EEG background activity is present. There is also an increase in respiratory rate and heart rate associated with this spell.

As previously discussed, nonspecific findings of hypersynchronous theta activity, theta-delta sleep, and hypersynchronous delta activity might be identified between spells. The most important diagnostic feature of these segments, however, is the technician's note in the record of the patient's behavior during the event. The technician noted that the "patient sat up suddenly/cry/panic look." This behavior was confirmed by review of the videotape segment that recorded the spell.

Polysomnography is indicated, only under certain circumstances, in children with symptoms of sleep terrors. These circumstances include situations where injury to the child is likely and the spells are associated with agitated sleep walking, thrashing, or violent movements; when spells are thought to be precipitated by other sleep-related disorders; when symptoms require differentiation from sleep-related seizure activity; and when medication is being considered as part of the therapeutic regimen.

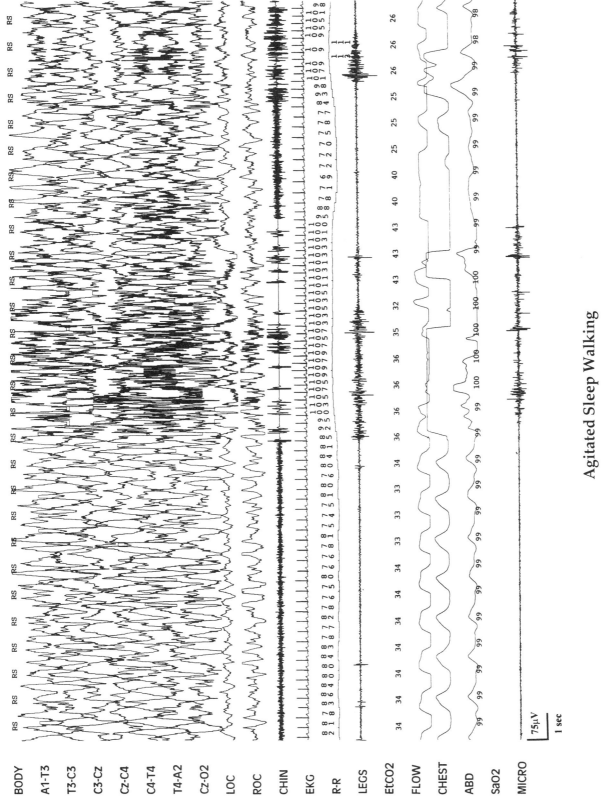

Agitated Sleep Walking

Figure 59. Agitated Sleep Walking

This 60-second epoch was recorded from a 10 1/2-year-old female who had a 5-year history of frantically running around the house, acting incoherently, and appearing to be in a panic state. Spells began approximately 1 hour after sleep onset and lasted about 5 minutes. There was rapid return to sleep and amnesia for the spells. Several injuries had occurred during the episodes. Note the sudden increase in muscle tone in the chin muscle EMG and anterior tibialis EMG associated with increased heart rate and irregular respiration. An arousal EEG rhythm, muscle artifact, and movement artifact are superimposed on a continuous background of high voltage slow waves at a frequency of approximately 0.5 Hz. Because of the prior injuries, 0.25 mg of lorazepam at bedtime was prescribed. Immediate resolution of symptoms occurred.

Agitated sleep walking is very similar to sleep terrors and may represent one of a continuum of symptoms related to NREM partial arousal disorders. Agitated sleep walking differs from sleep terrors in that with agitated sleep walking there is displacement from the bed. During a spell, children will get out of bed and behave in a confused and disoriented manner and they may run around the home in an apparent panic state. Injury can occur with these disorders, although the exact frequency is unknown. Children may run into walls or doors, or they may fall down stairs. They may perform complex activities during episodes of agitated sleep walking, and, at these times they are quite difficult to awaken and comfort. As with other NREM motor disorders, etiology appears to be maturational, and spontaneous resolution is typical. Medical treatment is indicated only when there is considerable risk of injury or there is significant family disruption from the spells. In most cases, behavioral interventions should be attempted prior to institution of medicinal therapy.

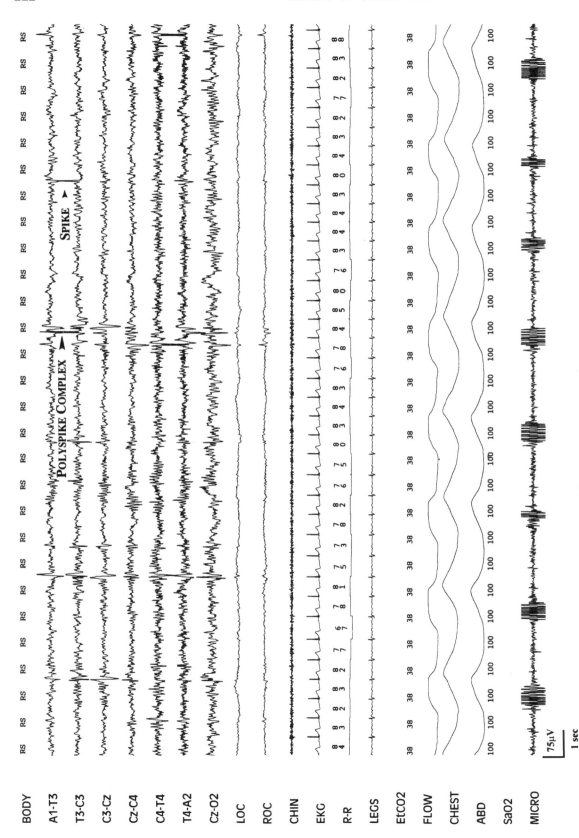

Episodic Nocturnal Wanderings

Figure 60a. Episodic Nocturnal Wanderings

The polysomnographic epochs shown in Figures 60a and 60b were recorded from a 15-year-old patient with a history suggestive of agitated sleep walking and automatic, repetitive behaviors during sleep. Attacks occurred several times per night and were associated with violent behavior. There was no family history of parasomnias, but there was a younger brother had a history of generalized tonic-clonic seizures.

Figure 60a reveals frequent multifocal independent spike and polyspike activity in the standard polysomnogram montage.

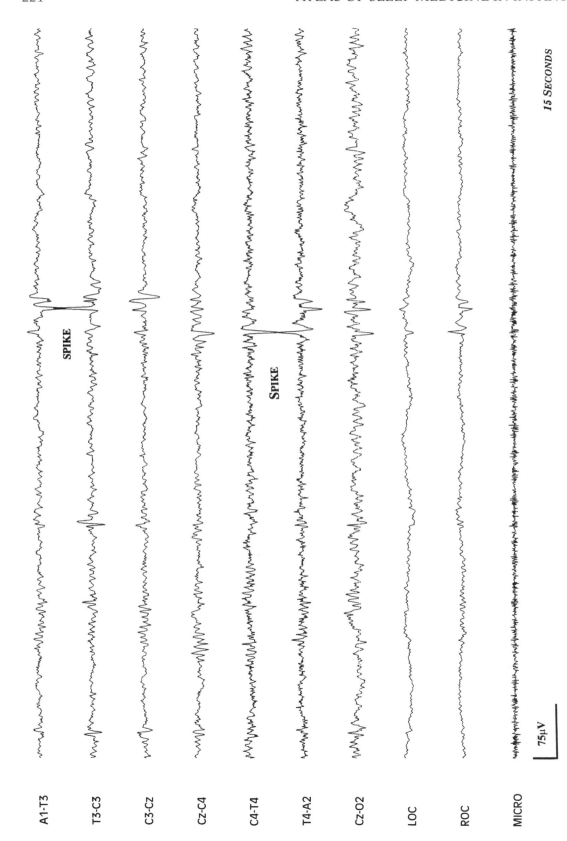

Episodic Nocturnal Wanderings

Figure 60b. Episodic Nocturnal Wanderings

This figure shows a 15-second segment of EEG, EOG, and chin muscle EMG, clearly revealing the different hemispheric fields of epileptiform activity. This patient responded well to carbamazepine. Symptoms decreased to one episode per year. Symptoms returned after a trial of weaning from medication. Re-institution of the anti-convulsant medication again resulted in resolution of symptoms.

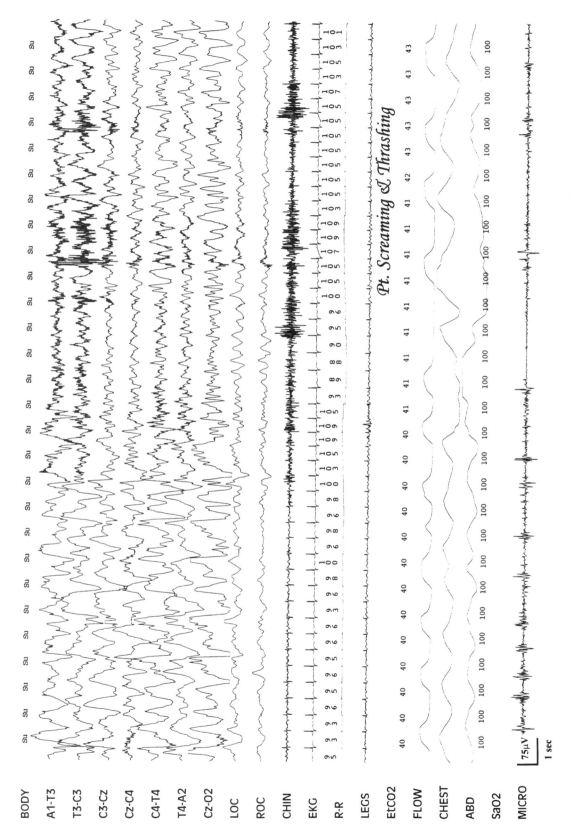

Confusional Arousals

Figure 61. Confusional Arousals

This 30-second polysomnographic segment was recorded from a 13-year-old male with a history of frequent disorientation and violent behavior upon being awakened for school each morning. Note the partial arousal from SWS. EEG background activity is replaced by a faster waking background rhythm, yet screaming and thrashing is documented. The patient was eventually comforted by his parent after a short period (less than 2 minutes during this episode in the laboratory), and remained awake and frightened for approximately 30 minutes. No dreams were reported.

Confusional arousals are similar to other partial arousal parasomnias. Arousal, however, seems to occur to a higher level of alertness and the patient often remembers the event. Upon arousal, the child is confused, disoriented, and often frightened. Symptoms may occur after the patient is awakened from a somnambulistic attack. At times, confusion and disorientation is profound and it may be difficult to comfort the patient. Confusional arousals may be precipitated by attempts to awaken children from slow-wave sleep or may occur independently due to internal arousal mechanisms.

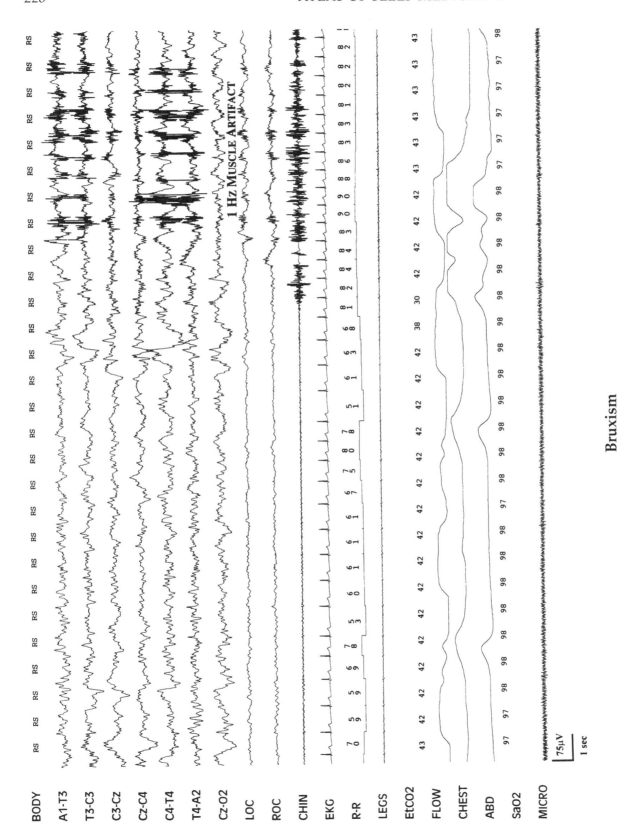

Bruxism

Figure 62. Bruxism

This polysomnogram epoch was recorded from a 9-year-old female who complained of headaches upon awakening each morning. Rhythmic, 1-Hz muscle artifact is recorded in the EEG channels and chin muscle EMG. This episode of bruxism occurred during an arousal from stage 2 sleep. Note the relatively low voltage, mixed frequency EEG background activity and sleep spindles prior to the arousal and bruxism. Rhythmic muscle artifact appears symmetrically over the temporalis muscle on each side of the head. Because of the placement of EOG electrodes in close proximity to the origin of the anterior portion of the temporalis muscle, rhythmic muscle artifact can also be seen in LOC and ROC.

Bruxism is common during childhood and can present in a variety of ways. Grinding of teeth may be associated with loud, highly disagreeable sound. At other times, it may be associated with vigorous rhythmic clenching of teeth without the generation of sound. Bruxism can be seen during any NREM sleep stage and during wakefulness. It typically does not occur during REM sleep due to active inhibition of skeletal muscle tone.

Patients may complain of nocturnal waking with headaches, temporomandibular joint problems, morning cephalgia, wearing down of the crowns of teeth, or any combination of these symptoms. Parents often complain of the noxious noise, which keeps them awake at night.

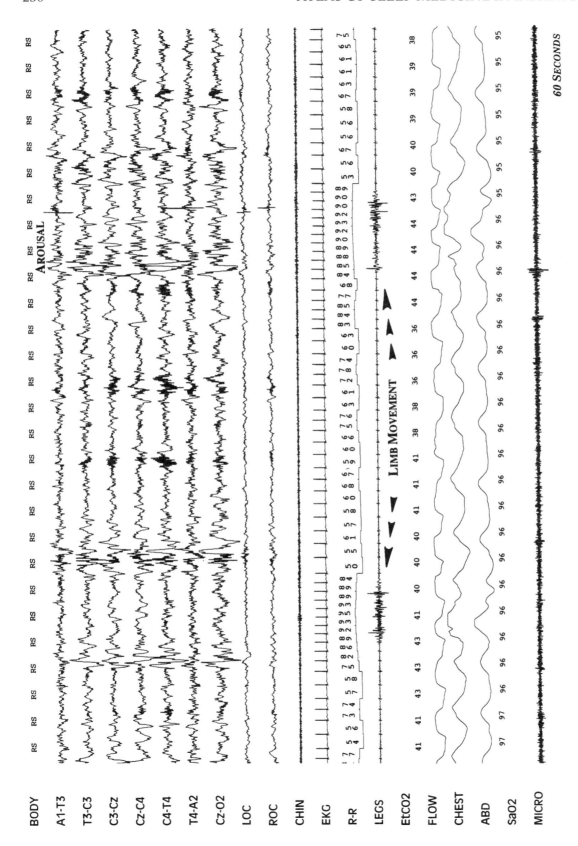

Periodic Limb Movement Disorder

Figure 63a. Periodic Limb Movement Disorder

The polysomnographic epochs in Figures 63a through 63c were recorded from a 6½-year-old female who had a history of restless sleep, daytime hyperactivity alternating with somnolence, learning problems, and behavioral difficulties in school. Her attention span was very poor, and her mother reported the girl was always fidgety.

Figure 63a is a *60-second* segment recorded during stage 2 sleep. Characteristic limb movements are present in the bilaterally linked anterior tibialis EMG. Muscle tone waxes and wanes, resulting in a characteristic *capsule.* Leg movements are followed by approximately 4 to 5 seconds of 6- to 7-Hz EEG activity representing an arousal rhythm. Respiration and heart rate both increase with each arousal.

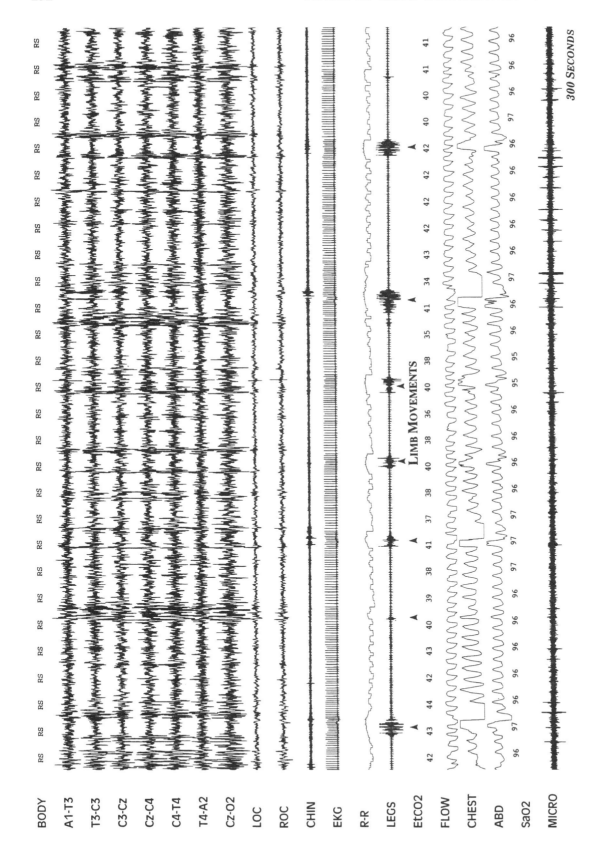

Periodic Limb Movement Disorder

Figure 63b. Periodic Limb Movement Disorder

This segment represents *300 seconds* of recording in the same patient, and demonstrates periodicity of the limb movements as well as fragmentation of sleep continuity by brief movement and/or electrocortical arousals.

Periodic limb movement disorder is thought to be unusual in young children. Exact prevalence is unknown, but it seems to be more common if there is a strong family history of this disorder. Treatment is based on comprehensive clinical evaluation and severity of daytime and nocturnal symptoms. Patients should be closely monitored. This patient responded very well to small doses of clonazepam (0.25 mg) 30 minutes prior to bedtime.

Nocturnal symptoms might include restless sleep, leg and/or arm twitching, and limb movements during sleep. Occasionally, there are frequent arousals and awakenings from stage 2 sleep. At other times there may be partial arousals from SWS. Little is known about periodic limb movement disorder in children. Based on clinical observations, periodic movements of the arms can be seen in some children, and sometimes precede leg movements. Finally, limb movements may not fulfill all criteria required for diagnosis in the adult patient, as limb movements will often result in an awakening or major body movement.

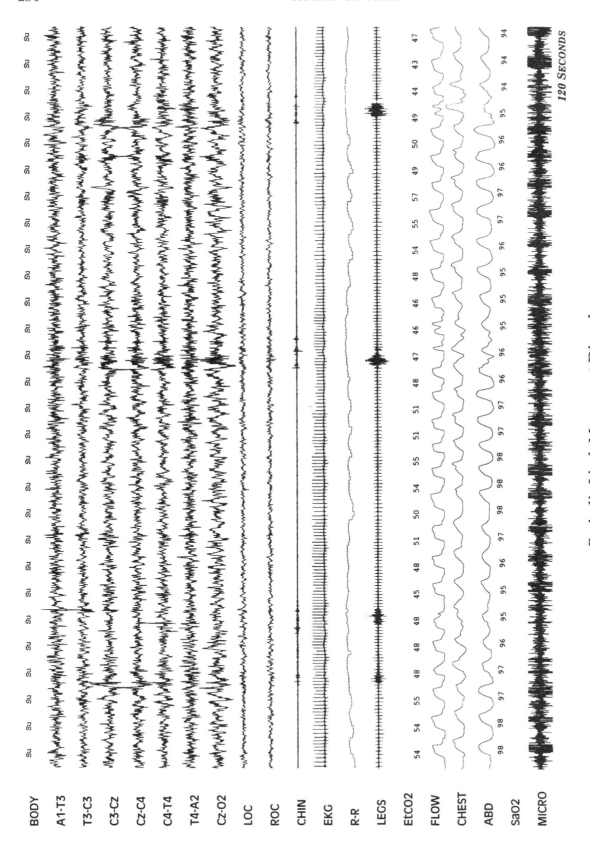

Periodic Limb Movement Disorder

Figure 63c. Periodic Limb Movement Disorder

This figure shows a recording from a 6-year-old male with a history of hyperactivity, daytime sleepiness on weekends, and poor school performance. There was a history of mild snoring, but the child's mother stated that the snoring was only mild and occurred when the boy had a "cold." There was a narrow nasal airway and tonsils were hypertrophied.

It is often difficult to evaluate the significance of periodic limb movements recorded polysomnographically in children. Movements may be associated with arousal secondary to high upper airway resistance and occult partially occlusive respiratory events. In this 120-second polysomnographic segment, note arousal immediately *preceding* the leg movements and preceding the persistently elevated E_tCO_2, suggesting obstructive hypoventilation secondary to high upper airway resistance.

In addition to patient-related phenomena, we have also recorded similar fragmentation of the continuity of sleep associated with limb movements and brief arousals in young children in the laboratory, due to environmental factors. Parents typically "room in" with their children in the sleep laboratory. Some parents have been noted to snore loudly during sleep. Parental snoring is associated with pauses and snorts suggestive of obstructive sleep apnea syndrome. The children often arouse with each parental snort. Technician documentation and environmental control is essential for controlling this environmental artifact (obstructive sleep apnea syndrome by proxy).

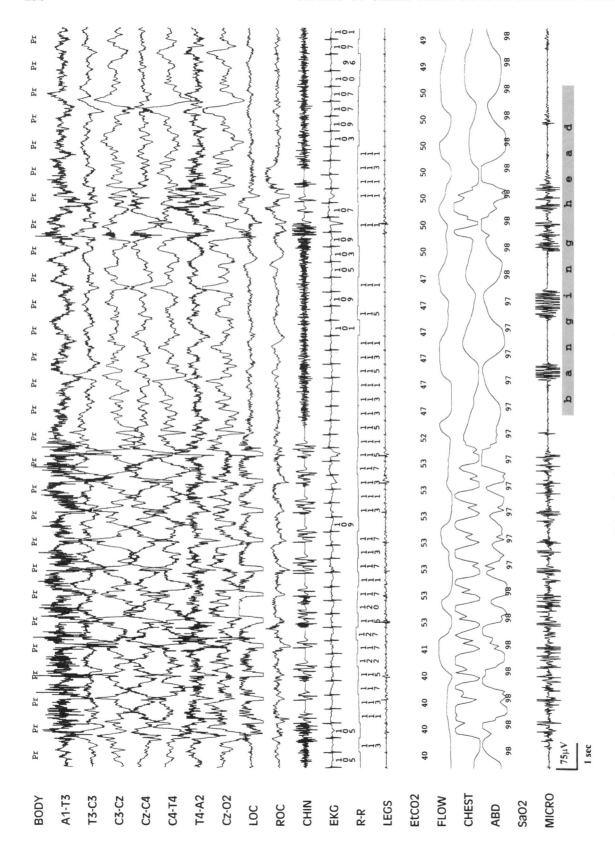

Rhythmic Movement Disorders

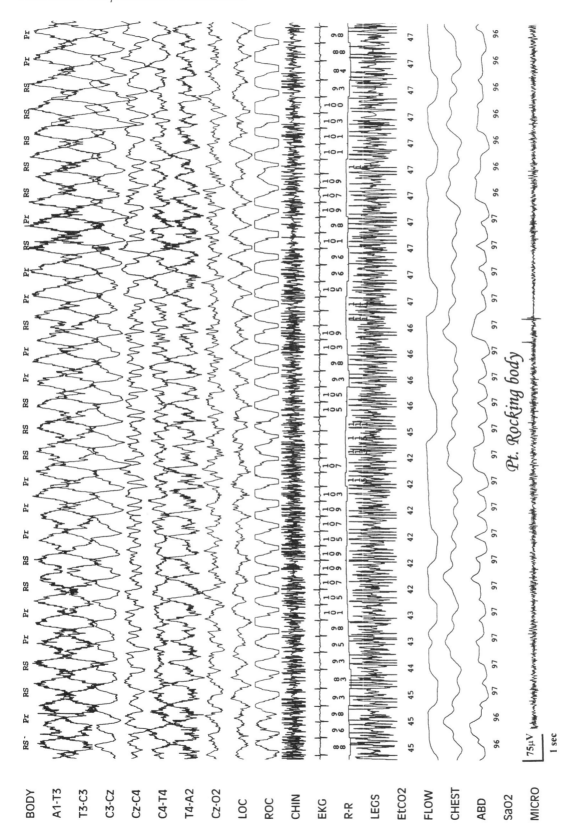

Pt. Rocking body

Rhythmic Movement Disorders, *continued*

Figures 64a and 64b. Rhythmic Movement Disorders

The polysomnographic segments shown in Figures 64a and 64b were recorded from a 3-year-old female who had a history of head banging while falling asleep and during sleep. She was otherwise well. The history was negative for seizures, and physical examination was normal except for several small bruises on her forehead.

Figure 64a was recorded during SWS. Note the rhythmic muscle artifact obscuring the first 10 seconds of the recording. Episodes of head banging were documented by video several times during the polysomnogram, and the technician noted rhythmic head banging and body rocking (Figure 64b) on the record.

Jactatio capitis nocturnes (nocturnal head banging) most commonly occurs during the period just prior to sleep onset, during wake-to-sleep transitions. It typically persists into transitional stage 1 sleep and ceases with sleep onset. It rarely occurs during SWS. Rhythmic head banging is rare during REM sleep. Occasionally, this sleep-wake transition disorder can occur during NREM sleep (stage 2 or SWS) and after arousals. When severe, quality of life is disturbed for both the patient and his or her entire family. Although injury is rare, rhythmic head banging can be quite violent, resulting in superficial contusions and occasionally lacerations. Rhythmic head banging may also be associated with other rhythmic movements of the head and body, including body shuttling and rhythmic head rolling. Rhythmic movement of extremities is rarely involved. When rhythmic, paroxysmal movements involve arms and legs, seizure disorder and hypnogenic paroxysmal dystonia must be included in the differential diagnosis.

Part 3

REM Sleep-Related Parasomnias

The majority of parasomnias that occur during childhood are related to NREM sleep. Some parasomnias, however, are characteristically present during REM sleep. These include nightmares and REM-sleep motor disorder (known as REM-sleep behavior disorder, or RBD, in adults). Both must be clinically and polysomnographically differentiated from NREM motor parasomnias and other anxiety-related sleep disorders. Clinical symptoms can be overlapping and may appear remarkably similar. Often, parents may describe sleep terrors as severe nightmares, and nightmares may be described as frequent night wakings. Although these disorderes are clinically and pathophysiologically different, parent/caretaker *interpretation* of sleep-related behaviors may not provide enough information to differentiate between the two. Careful analysis in the clinic will often provide enough information to differentiate these disorders, and a clinical trial of behavioral treat-ment is most often warranted prior to polysomnography. Polysomnography should be considered in order to assist in differentiation under one or more of the following conditions: when initial interventions fail to result in symptom resolution, when there is a high risk of injury, when medication is being considered, or when other portions of the clinical evaluation indicate. Although polysomnography is rarely required, it may occasionally be needed for accurate diagnosis.

Suggested Reading

1. Ross RJ, Ball WA, Dinges DF, et al: Motor dysfunction during sleep in post-traumatic stress disorder. Sleep 1994;17:723–732.
2. Sheldon SH, Jacobsen J: REM-sleep motor disorder in children. J Child Neurol 1998;13:257–260.

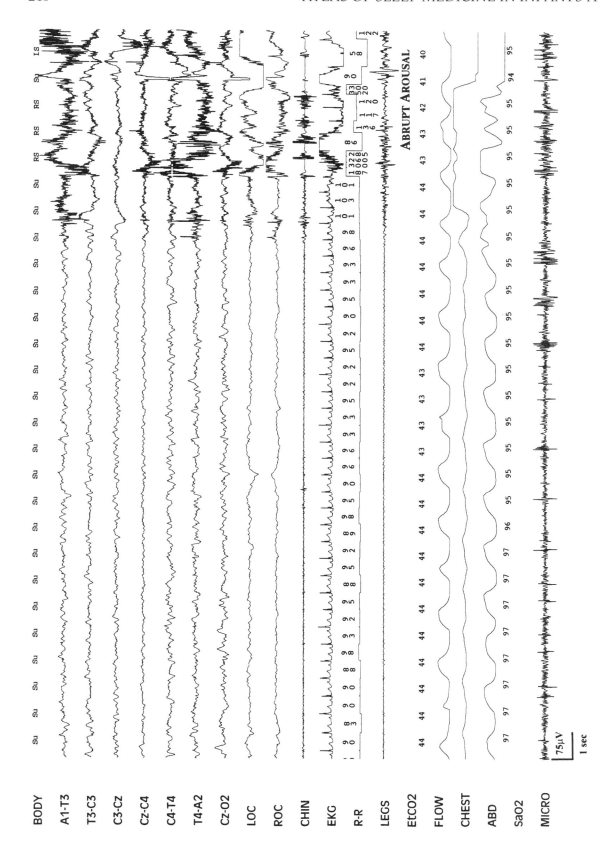

Nightmares

Figure 65. Nightmares

This polysomnographic epoch was recorded during REM sleep from a 5-year-old female who was referred for evaluation of snoring. On initial clinic consultation, parents reported frequent early morning wakings and vivid nightmares occurring two to three times per week. The patient had some difficulty in settling at the beginning of her sleep period, but once asleep she remained asleep until about 03:00.

In the laboratory, the patient demonstrated an abrupt arousal and awakening from REM sleep. After this awakening she exhibited mild agitation and fear. She related a vivid dream of being chased through her house by her older brother. She was easily comforted by her mother after the episode, but return to sleep was somewhat prolonged. Heart rate is mildly elevated during the arousal, but no other symptoms suggesting increased autonomic activity are present.

This is a classic presentation of nightmares, and it demonstrates features that differentiate these anxiety dreams from sleep terrors. Sleep terrors arise abruptly from SWS. In contrast, nightmares occur out of REM sleep and are typically associated with vivid recall of the anxiety-provoking dream. Autonomic activity is much milder during a nightmare than an NREM sleep terror. The youngster is almost always easily soothed by the caretaker after a nightmare, and return to sleep is prolonged.

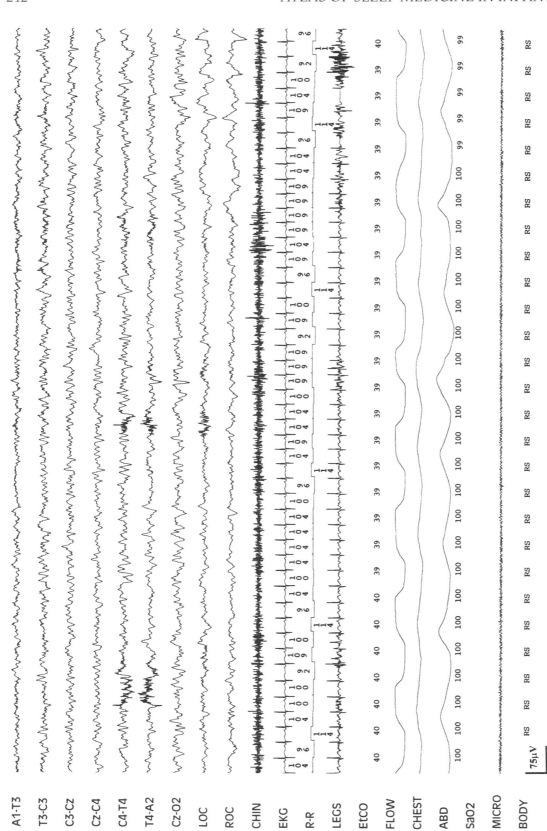

REM-Sleep Motor Disorder/REM-Sleep Behavior Disorder

Figure 66. REM-Sleep Motor Disorder/REM-Sleep Behavior Disorder

This 30-second polysomnographic segment was recorded from a 6-year-old male with a history of "fighting in his sleep." He had fractured two metatarsal bones after kicking the headboard of his bed. Characteristics of REM-sleep behavior disorder (RBD) are present. The term REM-sleep motor disorder (RMD) has been used because it may more accurately describe the physiological state dissociation occurring in this syndrome. In this REM sleep epoch, chin muscle tone is increased, major body movements are present, and vocalizations occur without state change. Increased periodic and intermittent limb movements can be seen. Major body and limb movements have been shown to occur in children with RMD when compared to a control group.

Symptoms of RMD can range from a variety of motor activities to automatic behaviors associated with vivid dream mentation. Displacement from bed has been reported, and significant injury can occur. As in adult patients with RBD, response to treatment with clonazepam is rapid and symptoms are typically well controlled. In a study by Ross and co-workers, adult patients with post-traumatic stress disorder (PTSD) can present with similar polysomnographic findings. Interestingly, in a preliminary retrospective analysis of 23 children who were victims of physical and/or sexual abuse and were diagnosed with PTSD, similar findings were present. These interesting observations require prospective and systematic study.

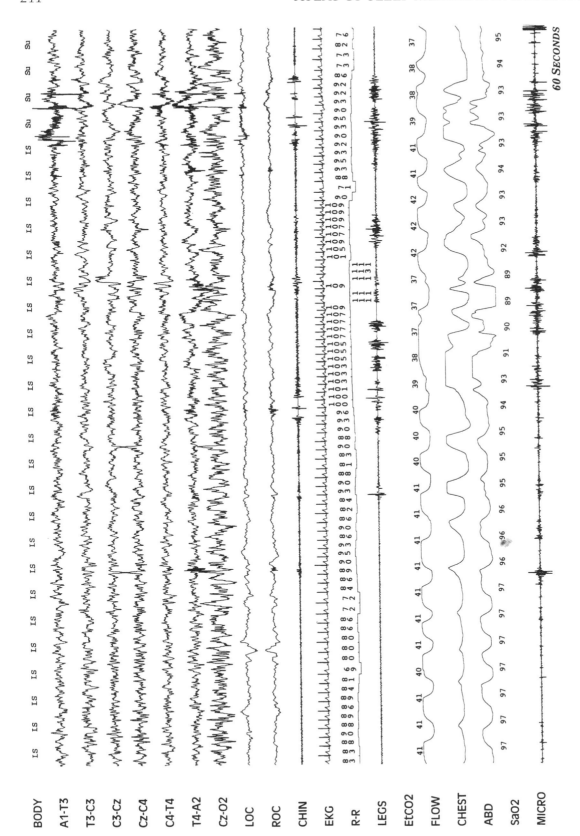

Post-Traumatic Stress Disorder (PTSD)

Figure 67. Post-Traumatic Stress Disorder (PTSD)

This *60-second* polysomnographic segment was recorded from a 5-year-old female who had suffered severe burn injuries and smoke inhalation during a fire in her home. She had been hospitalized for approximately 3 months in a burn unit and for 8 months in a rehabilitation hospital. Upon returning home, she experienced severe recurrent nightmares and clinical depression. Episodes of screaming, yelling, and thrashing about in bed occurred nightly. Vivid dreams of "batting at flames" in front of her face were reported. Sleep onset after lights-out was prolonged. Full awakenings followed episodes of screaming. Once awake, she was easily soothed by her parents, but return to sleep ranged from 60 to 120 minutes. Daytime sleepiness was reported, but the youngster refused napping, stating she was "afraid to fall asleep."

This segment demonstrates increased chin muscle tone with excessive phasic activity during REM sleep. There are periods of paradoxical increased muscle tone, clear EEG characteristics of REM sleep with a relatively low voltage, mixed frequency background, and trains of sawtooth waves. These polysomnographic findings must be differentiated from body movements associated with nightmares.

Little is known regarding polysomnographic findings in children with PTSD. Limited polysomnographic data are available in adults. Ross observed increased phasic activity, increased muscle tone, and increased periodic limb movement in adult Vietnam veterans diagnosed with PTSD. Our observations are similar, however further systematic testing and replication is required.

Part 4

Sleep in the Neurologically Challenged Child

Disordered sleep is common in children who are neurologically challenged. A variety of problems exist and symptoms may reflect disorders related to cortical function, subcortical function, and/or lower brain stem function. Sleep-disordered breathing is common in children with neurological disabilities, especially if pharyngeal muscle activity is affected by the disorder. Although previously covered in detail, sleep-related breathing disorders are presented in this section only as they relate to the child's underlying neurological abnormality.

Sleep-wake schedule problems are also common in patients with central neurological disabilities. Circadian rhythm abnormalities frequently occur and may be better assessed using actigraphic recordings rather than polysomnography.

Sleep-related seizure disorders are common. Sleeping state is a potent activator of epileptic seizure activity. Frequently, seizure activity is best identified during sleep. At times a circadian increase in seizure activity can be seen during the major sleep period. Comprehensive polysomnography with an expanded EEG electrode array is an ideal procedure to screen for many epileptic disorders. Included in this section are polysomnographic segments demonstrating a number of epileptiform abnormalities which can be identified and assessed in the sleep laboratory. Some are common, others unusual. Depicted segments have been recorded at standard polysomnogram speed of 30 mm per second, resulting in 30-second epochs. They are also presented in 15-second epochs, which more closely approximate standard EEG recording speed.

Spikes, sharp waves, and polyspike discharges can often be identified on polysomnographic epochs. A *sharp transient* is an event which clearly stands out against the EEG background and has a pointed peak at standard EEG speed. A *sharp wave* is a sharp transient with a duration of 70 to 200 ms, and a *spike* is a sharp transient with a duration of 20 to 70 ms. A *polyspike discharge* is a polyphasic spike with two or more components occurring on opposite sides of the baseline. Spikes and sharp waves, which rarely occur during a recording or recur with varying morphology, are often termed *sharp transients* because they have less significance in the diagnosis of seizure disorders than stereotypic waveforms.

Although many disabling neurological conditions associated with disordered sleep are secondary to the underlying central nervous system disease process, identification and management of the sleep-related abnormality may affect the patient and family in a number of important ways. First, the sleep disorder may contribute to the underlying central nervous system disability, exacerbating the condition. Second, the sleep disorder may result in daytime symptoms, thereby undermining rehabilitative interventions. Finally, improving sleep may improve quality of life for the entire family, even though there may be no primary effect on the patient's underlying neurological condition.

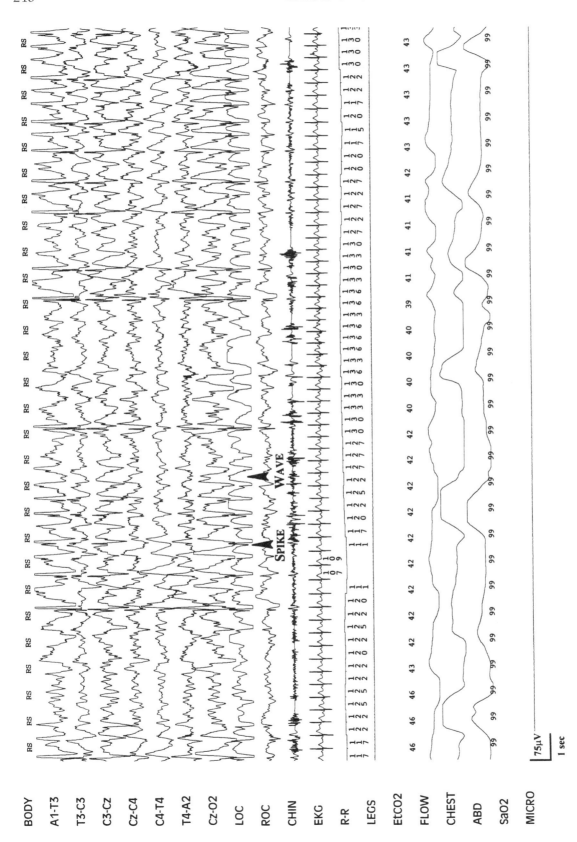

Continuous Generalized Spike-and-Wave Discharges of Sleep

Figure 68. Continuous Generalized Spike-and-Wave Discharges of Sleep

This 30-second polysomnogram segment was recorded from a 5-year-old female with spastic quadriplegia secondary to anoxic encephalopathy. Clinical seizures had been well controlled with phenytoin. Frequency of the spike-and-wave discharges is about 0.5 to 1.0 Hz, and the continuous epileptiform activity made scoring of NREM sleep difficult. Greatest activity seems to be located over the left hemisphere, but both right and left hemispheric involvement is present. Also note the appearance of spike-and-wave activity in the left eye channel, with minimal activity seen in the right eye channel. Interestingly, the $Cz-O_2$ scoring channel reveals minimal abnormal electrical activity. If a more limited EEG recording were done in this patient, the significance of this EEG abnormality might have been overlooked. Technician documentation and video recording of motor movements (or their absence) during electrical epileptiform activity is important in evaluation. Absence of increased heart rate or changes in respiratory pattern suggests an electrical abnormality and not seizure activity.

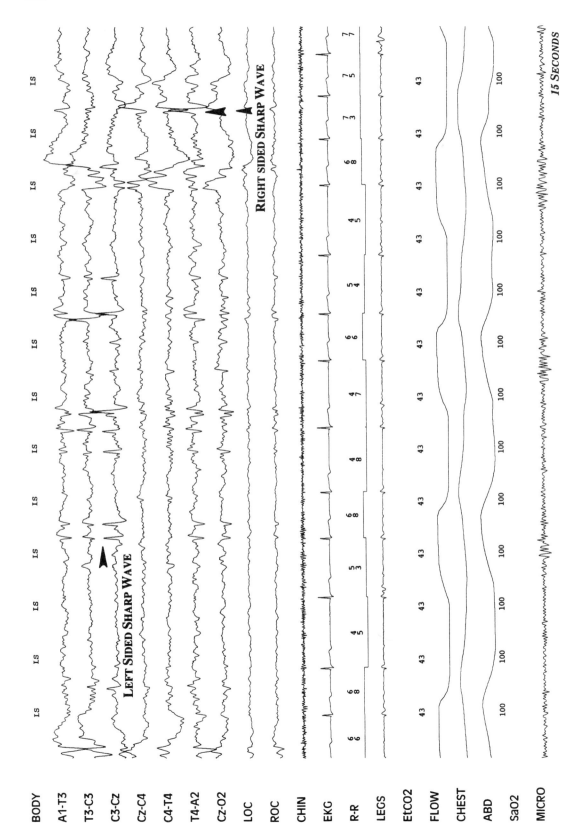

Bi-Temporal Spikes and Sharp Waves

Figure 69. Bi-Temporal Spikes and Sharp Waves

This 15-second polysomnographic segment was recorded from a 7-year-old male who presented with a history of loud snoring associated with pauses and snorts. There was a past history of partial complex seizures which had been treated with carbamazepine for 2 years. Clinical seizures resolved and the study was conducted to assess the patient for possible sleep-disordered breathing. Frequent synchronous and asynchronous bi-temporal sharp waves were noted during the recording. Spikes, polyspikes, and sharp waves are present. Note the apparent absence of epileptiform activity in the referential (Cz-O_2) channel. Heart rate is stable during the epoch. These spikes can be differentiated from EKG artifact by timing. Also, note snoring recorded in the sonogram. Oxygen saturation remains normal and E_tCO_2 is within normal limits.

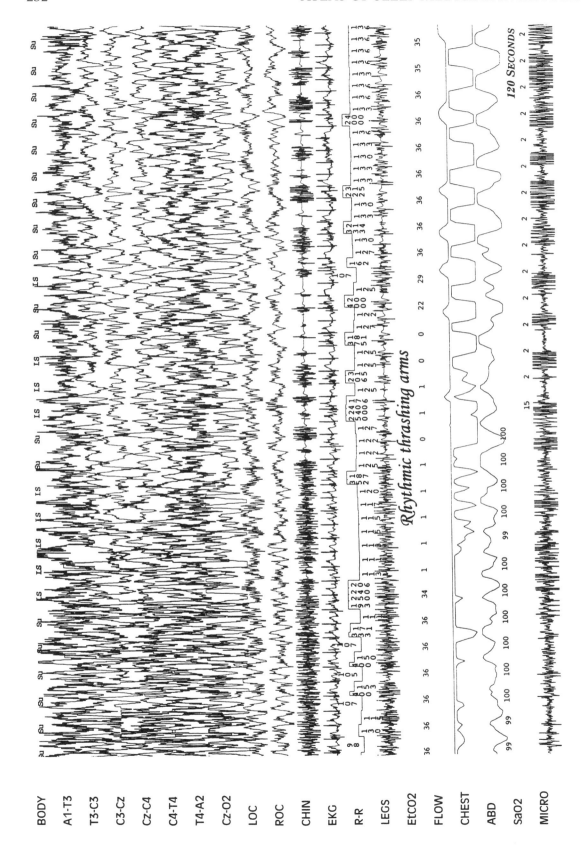

Hypnogenic Paroxysmal Dystonia

Figure 70a. Hypnogenic Paroxysmal Dystonia

The polysomnographic segments shown in Figures 70a and 70b were recorded from a 4-year-old female who presented for evaluation of unusual behaviors associated with rhythmic "flailing" movements of her arms and legs during sleep. Each night the patient rhythmically kicked her legs and thrashed about in bed. This behavior was very disturbing to her parents and it resulted in significant family disruption. Daytime function, performance, and development were otherwise normal. Comprehensive video-polysomnography was conducted.

Rhythmic thrashing of the arms and legs, associated with intermittent dystonic posturing of the hands and face suggested a diagnosis of hypnogenic paroxysmal dystonia. The child responded well to 50 mg of carbamazepine at bedtime.

Figure 70a demonstrates an abrupt arousal from SWS. There is sudden onset of movement artifact obscuring most of the recording. Artifact appears to be superimposed on a background of 0.5- to 1-Hz EEG activity. Respiratory rate is increased and a variable respiratory pattern is present. Oxygen saturation and E_tCO_2 remain normal. Vocalizations are noted by video and sonography.

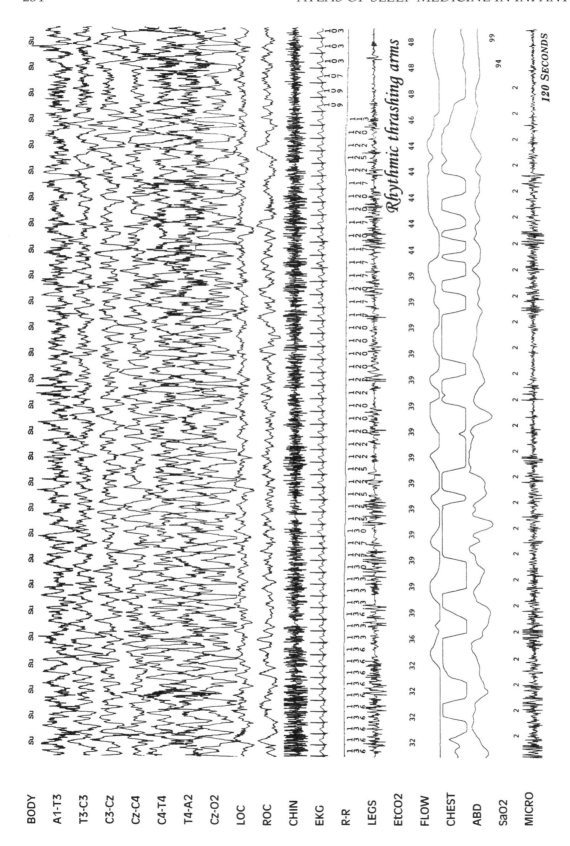

Hypnogenic Paroxysmal Dystonia

Figure 70b. Hypnogenic Paroxysmal Dystonia

The polysomnographic segment shown here demonstrates continued rhythmic kicking and shaking movements (as documented by video recording and technical notes). Gain, movement, and muscle artifact are superimposed on a slow-wave background EEG rhythm. Questionable sharp waves are noted in the EEG. A standard sleep-deprived EEG revealed no ictal abnormalities and an MRI of the patient's head was normal.

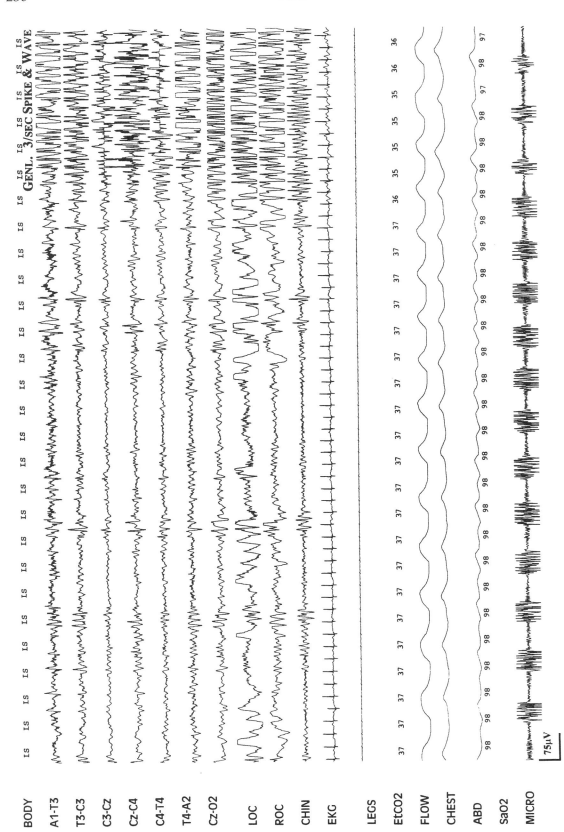

Three-per-Second Spike-and-Wave Activity

Figure 71a. Three-per-Second Spike-and-Wave Activity

The polysomnogram segments in Figures 71a through 71c were recorded from an 8-year-old male who presented with a history of school performance problems, behavioral problems, and day dreaming. Parents had noted brief staring spells during the day. There was a history of moderate snoring and unrefreshing sleep. Daytime sleepiness was common, yet the child rarely napped.

Figure 71a shows a 30-second epoch that was recorded during stage 2 sleep. Prior to this segment, there were questionable occasional left temporal spike-and-wave discharges. Snoring is clearly recorded in the sonogram. The patient is lying on his left side. E_tCO_2 and S_pO_2 are normal. During the last quarter of the epoch, there is an abrupt onset of continuous generalized three-per-second spike-and-wave activity.

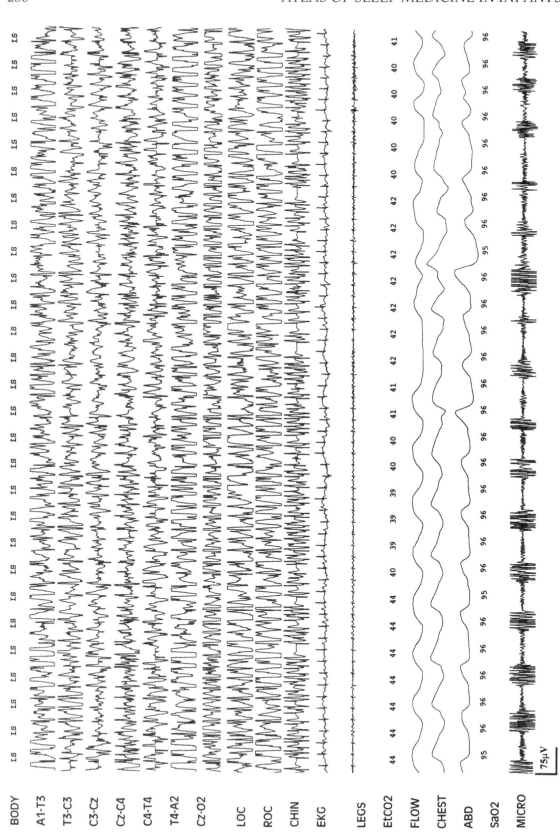

Three-per-Second Spike-and-Wave Activity

Figure 71b. Three-per-Second Spike-and-Wave Activity

This segment reveals continuous three-per-second spike-and-wave discharges which last about 45 seconds before spontaneous cessation. During this generalized epileptiform activity, there is no increase in heart rate or respiratory rate, suggesting the subclinical nature of this spell.

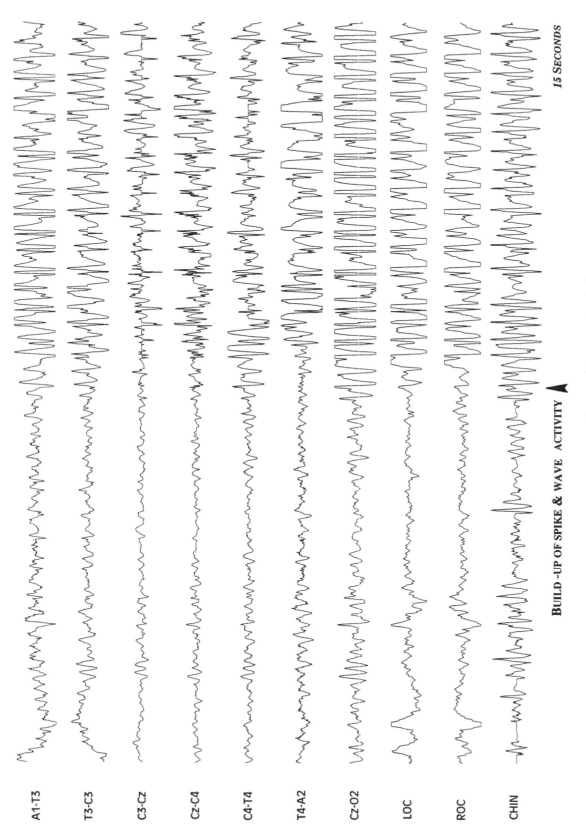

BUILD-UP OF SPIKE & WAVE ACTIVITY

Three-per-Second Spike-and-Wave Activity

15 SECONDS

Figure 71c. Three-per-Second Spike-and-Wave Activity

This figure depicts the onset of epileptiform activity in a *15-second* segment. Build-up of abnormal electrical activity can be seen immediately prior to the spell.

Partial complex seizure disorders are most frequently activated during sleep, and will most commonly occur during NREM stage 1 and stage 2 sleep. Electrical seizure activity is often attenuated during REM sleep and suppressed during wakefulness.

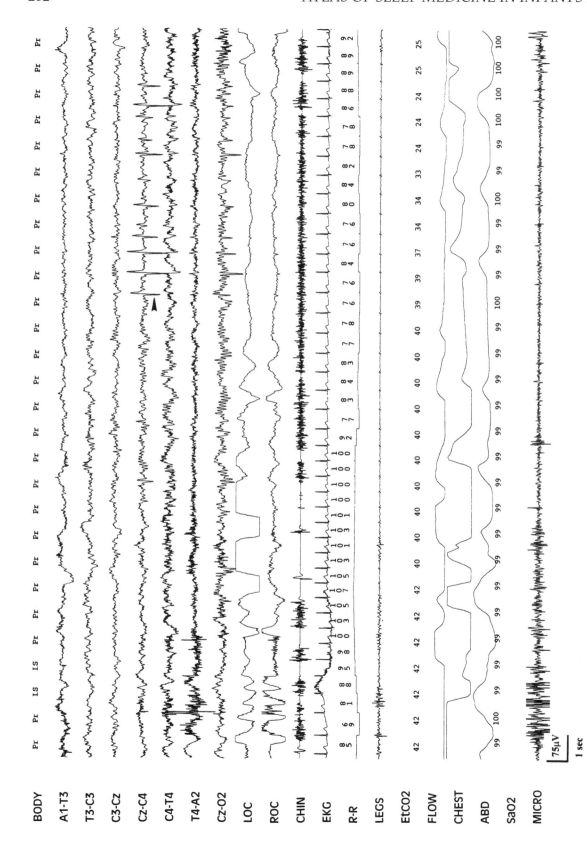

Unilateral Sharp Waves and Spikes

Figure 72a. Unilateral Sharp Waves and Spikes

The polysomnographic epochs shown in Figures 72a through 72c were recorded from a 4-year-old male under evaluation because of a history of loud snoring, restless sleep, daytime hyperactivity, and difficulty waking in the morning. Sleep architecture is normal. No significant sleep-disordered breathing was identified on this study. However, frequent right-sided sharp waves and spikes were present during wakefulness and sleep.

Figure 72a is a 30-second segment recorded during wakefulness. A predominant alpha rhythm can be seen in the EEG. High voltage right-sided spikes are present with a phase reversal over C4. Respiration, EKG, E_tCO_2, and S_pO_2 are normal. EKG artifact is unlikely, as these sharp transients are out of phase with the QRS complexes of the EKG (arrowheads).

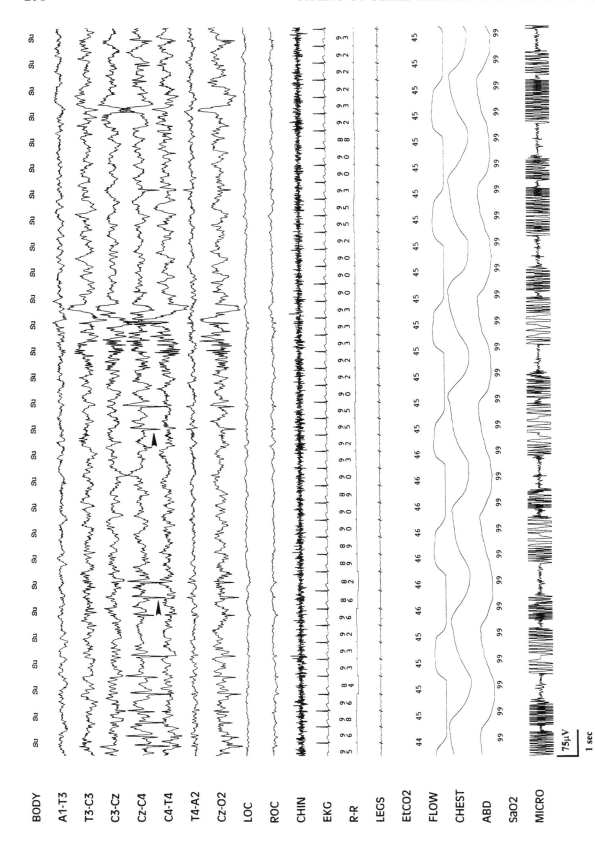

Unilateral Sharp Waves and Spikes

Figure 72b. Unilateral Sharp Waves and Spikes

Figure 72b shows a 30-second segment recorded during stage 2 sleep. K complexes and sleep spindles are present. Spikes are denoted by arrowheads.

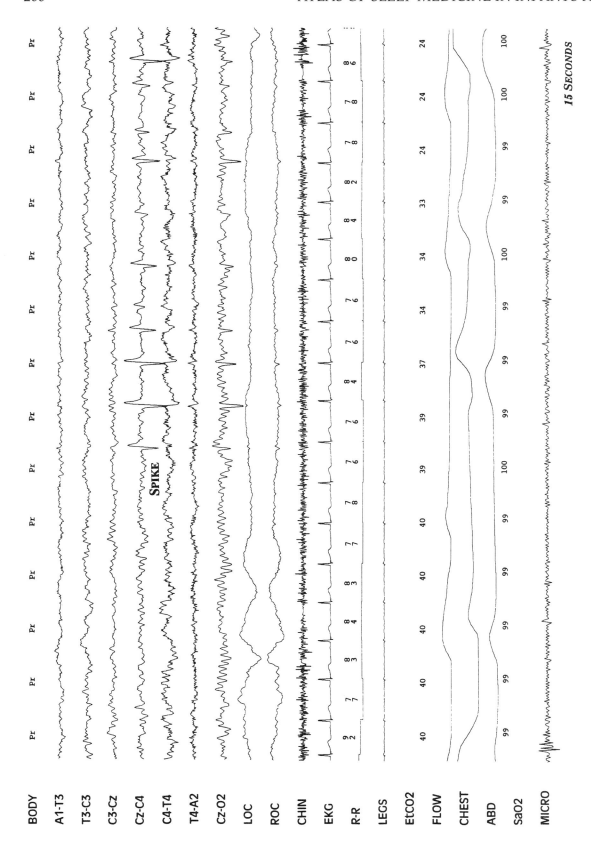

Unilateral Sharp Waves and Spikes

Figure 72c. Unilateral Sharp Waves and Spikes

This figure, a 15-second segment, now clearly shows the sharp nature of this electrical activity and a following wave resulting in a spike-and-wave complex.

These focal abnormalities of the EEG may represent *benign partial epilepsy of childhood with Rolandic spikes*. Onset is typically between 2 and 12 years of age and it typically disappears before or at puberty. No local brain lesions are identified, despite the clear focal nature of the EEG abnormality. Spikes are often followed by slow waves and tend to recur at rates of approximately 2 Hz. Location is usually centrotemporal and may be bilateral. Often partial seizures with simple motor symptoms may be present. Seizures are usually tonic or clonic, involve one side of the body, and may consist of cessation of speech. Secondary generalization is common. Seizures often occur at night and may go unnoticed unless they become generalized. A comprehensive sleep-deprived EEG and clinical neurological evaluation are required for accurate diagnosis.

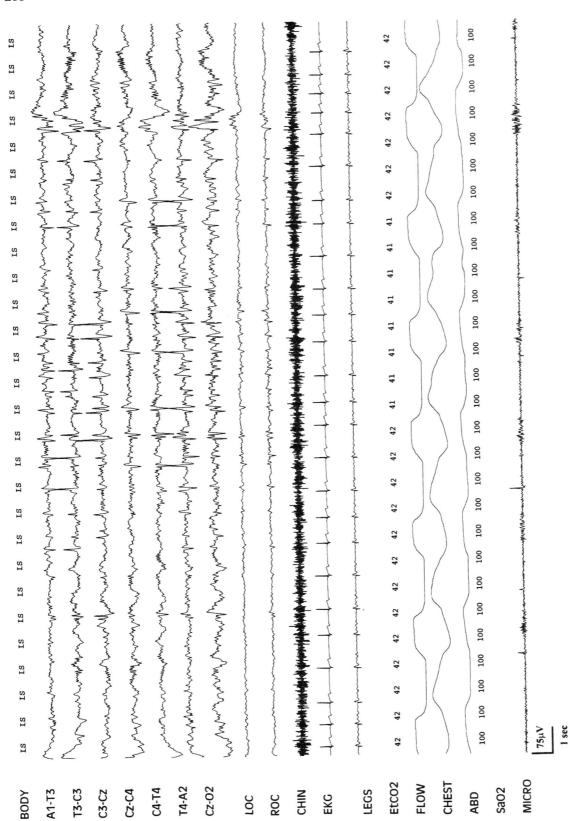

Multifocal Sharp Waves and Polyspike Discharges

Figure 73. Multifocal Sharp Waves and Polyspike Discharges

This 30-second polysomnographic epoch demonstrates multifocal, bilateral sharp waves and polyspike discharges recorded from an 8-year-old female with a history of spastic quadriplegia and generalized tonic-clonic seizures. Frequent independent left central spikes and polyspikes and right temporal sharp waves are depicted. The patient was experiencing sleep-wake cycle abnormalities and quality of life was disrupted for the patient's parents and siblings. EKG and respiration remained normal during NREM sleep, whereas significant REM-related obstructive apneas were present. Often, this epileptiform activity is attenuated during REM sleep and wakefulness. It is difficult, however, to relate the sleep-wake complaints and disorder with these epileptiform abnormalities. Indeed, they are most likely unrelated and both signs and symptoms are due to the child's underlying central nervous system disorder.

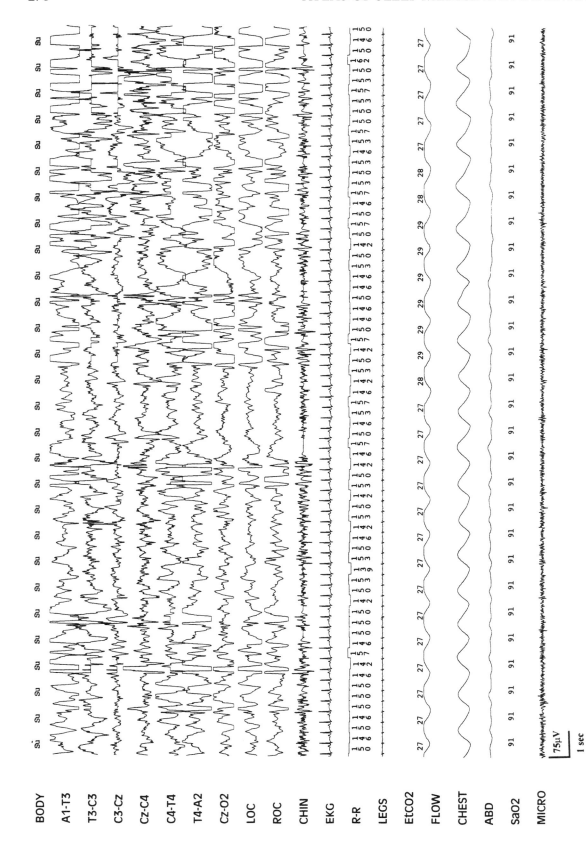

Hypsarrhythmia

BODY
A1-T3
T3-C3
C3-Cz
Cz-C4
C4-T4
T4-A2
Cz-O2
LOC
ROC
CHIN
EKG
R-R
LEGS
EtCO2
FLOW
CHEST
ABD
SaO2
MICRO

75μV

1 sec

Figure 74a. Hypsarrhythmia

Figure 74a represents a 30-second segment of an interesting polysomnogram recorded from an 8-month-old infant referred to the Pediatric Sleep Medicine Center for evaluation of an apparent life-threatening event and apnea associated with cyanosis. The patient's history was significant for meconium aspiration at birth and symptoms of infantile spasms. Diurnal EEG with complete electrode array revealed hypsarrhythmia. Nocturnal polysomnography revealed a similar EEG pattern. The patient was treated with ACTH with a good response in controlling clinical seizure symptoms. Again, it is most likely that the patient's clinical sleep-related symptoms and EEG abnormalities are unrelated and require separate approaches in management. However, ALTE may be due to sleep-related seizure activ-

ity, and polysomnography with an extended EEG electrode array should be considered as part of a comprehensive evaluation.

In these polysomnograms, no sleep spindles could be identified, no REM sleep was seen, and NREM sleep states could not be identified.

Technician comments are critical in determining sleep and wake states in polysomnograms such as these. Staging epochs in polysomnograms requires modification of standardized methods. Documenting wake and sleep may be all that is possible. State differentiation may not be necessary in interpretation of this polysomnogram, and clinical evaluation is of utmost importance. If REM sleep can be identified, it should be staged, but differentiation of NREM states is sometimes impossible.

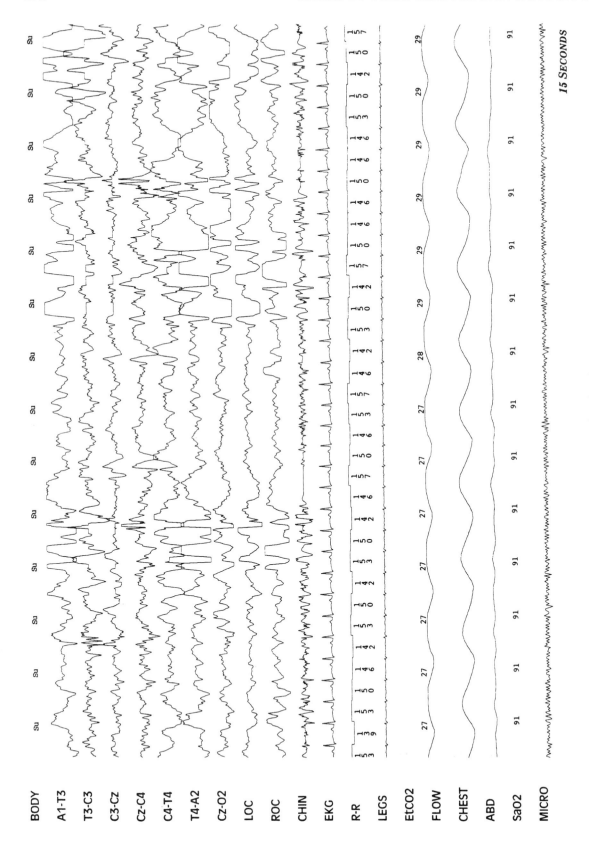

Hypsarrhythmia

15 Seconds

Figure 74b. Hypsarrhythmia
This figure shows a 15-second segment from the same 8-month-old patient.

Index